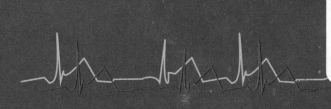

Understanding EKGs

A Practical Approach

FOURTH EDITION

BRENDA M. BEASLEY

MS, RN, EMT-Paramedic

09 · 44 · 14 · 44 75

PEARSON

Boston   Columbus   Indianapolis   New York   San Francisco   Upper Saddle River

Amsterdam   Cape Town   Dubai   London   Madrid   Milan   Munich   Paris   Montreal   Toronto

Delhi   Mexico City   São Paulo   Sydney   Hong Kong   Seoul   Singapore   Taipei   Tokyo

Publisher: Julie Levin Alexander
Publisher's Assistant: Regina Bruno
Editor-in-Chief: Marlene McHugh Pratt
Senior Acquisitions Editor: Sladjana Repic
Senior Managing Editor for Development: Lois Berlowitz
Editorial Assistant: Kelly Clark
Director of Marketing: David Gesell
Marketing Manager: Brian Hoehl
Marketing Specialist: Michael Sirinides
Marketing Assistant: Crystal Gonzalez

Managing Editor for Production: Patrick Walsh
Production Project Manager: Debbie Ryan
Editorial Project Manger: Patricia Guiterrez
Media Project Manager: Lorena Cerisano
Art Director: Jayne Conte
Cover Designer: Suzanne Behnke
Cover Image: Brenda M. Beasley
Composition: Aptara®, Inc.
Printer/Binder: Courier/Kendalville
Cover Printer: LeHigh-Phoenix Color/Hagerstown

Credits and acknowledgments borrowed from other sources and reproduced, with permission, in this textbook appear on the appropriate page within text.

Notice: The author and the publisher of this book have taken care to make certain that the information given is correct and compatible with the standards generally accepted at the time of publication. Nevertheless, as new information becomes available, changes in treatment and in the use of equipment and procedures become necessary. The reader is advised to carefully consult the instruction and information material included in each piece of equipment or device before administration. Students are warned that the use of any techniques must be authorized by their medical advisor, where appropriate, in accordance with local laws and regulations. The author and the publisher disclaim any liability, loss, injury, or damage incurred as a consequence, directly or indirectly, of the use and application of any of the contents of this book.

Many of the designations by manufacturers and sellers to distinguish their products are claimed as trademarks. Where those designations appear in this book, and the publisher was aware of a trademark claim, the designations have been printed in initial caps or all caps.

Library of Congress Cataloging-in-Publication Data

Beasley, Brenda M.
   Understanding EKGs : a practical approach / Brenda M. Beasley, MS, RN, EMT-Paramedic.—Fourth edition.
      pages cm
   Includes index.
   ISBN-13: 978-0-13-314772-8
   ISBN-10: 0-13-314772-X
   1. Electrocardiography.   I. Title.
   RC683.5.E5B378 2014
   616.1'207547—dc23   2013011016

10 9 8 7 6 5 4 3 2 1

PEARSON

ISBN 13: 978-0-13-314772-8
ISBN 10:   0-13-314772-X

Dedication

This book is dedicated to my precious children, David & Kathy Beasley and Paul & Melanie Skvarek, and my grandchildren, Lauren, Jonathan, Mariah, Emilio, Jessica, Will, Malachi, Nehemiah, Casey and Nicole. "You may not be from my body, but you will always be a part of my heart. I love you all very much."

and

to Michael C. West, MS, RN, EMT-P

Your assistance, support, encouragement, and constancy were invaluable to me throughout this revision process, and I am very grateful for, and blessed by, your friendship,

and

to the memory of my parents, Mr. and Mrs. Jack Messer—my role models for life.

Brief Contents

Detailed Contents

Foreword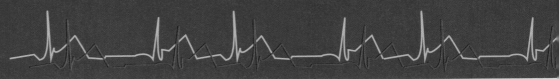

Dr. Willis D. Israel, who was my mentor and dear friend, has now departed this earth for a better place. His invaluable advice and wisdom were indispensable to me throughout my life, both personally and professionally. As a tribute to him, for always being there for me and for expecting and demanding the very best of me, the Foreword that was written by him for the original manuscript of this book is included in this edition.

When advanced life-support training for paramedical personnel was still considered questionable by most of my physician colleagues, I became involved in teaching advanced cardiac life support (ACLS). It soon became apparent that emergency medical technicians—in those days very frequently volunteer and/or part-time workers in the field—were frequently the most enthusiastic and responsive students of ACLS. Their eagerness to learn and to provide the whole range of prehospital care has proved to be a huge factor in patient survival.

I loved every moment I taught ACLS (as well as BCLS, emergency medical technician training, and advanced trauma life support)—whether to physicians, nurses, or paramedical personnel. Indeed, the teachers of these basic and extremely important concepts have impacted all areas of current medical care. Many of those with whom I taught ACLS became my close and greatly cherished friends. One of these is Brenda Messer Beasley, MS, RN, EMT-P, with whom I shared in teaching the first EMT course ever offered in rural Randolph County, Alabama. From the initial class session, I saw that Ms. Beasley had an extraordinary ability to render a complicated concept in its most basic form of expression. Though she had this gift for rendering the complex in simple terms, she never allowed the importance of what she was teaching to be lost, and she always stressed the awareness of and evaluation of the patient.

Ms. Beasley brings to this text on EKG interpretation the same ability to simplify the complex for the health care professional. Real meaning is surely more valuable than the easy "information overload" encountered when we deal with real patients in a medical emergency.

After I had taught with Ms. Beasley, she made a career change from nursing to full-time EMT training, still in our same basic geographical area. It became fun and rewarding as a practicing small-town family physician to be aware of prehospital care that had been rendered by students of this teacher. Their expertise was (is) impressive, as was their attention to the care of and the state of the patient. Certainly, any physician's ability to treat, and any patient's ultimate well-being, depends greatly on that initial prehospital care.

An appropriate text on EKG interpretation can only deepen the perception and understanding of the health care professional; at the same time, this text seems to teach and reteach the basic concept from every situation: "First, look at your patient, and continue to look at your patient."

I am honored to welcome this book to the plentiful material available on the heart, its functions, the circulatory system and its signals of dysfunction and illness.

Willis D. Israel, MD
Wedowee, AL

Preface

This informative and simple approach to EKG analysis continues in this, the fourth edition of this textbook. Based on the fact that cardiology and basic EKG interpretation are integral parts of most primary and allied health-related curricula, I originally wrote this book to assist the novice student in his or her understanding of basic EKG interpretation, and that purpose remains undaunted. This book is intended for the health care provider at the initial level(s) of understanding of cardiovascular anatomy, physiology, and rhythm strip interpretation. The categories of students who will benefit from this text include pre-hospital care providers, medical students, cardiac care monitor techs, ACLS candidates, nursing professionals, physician assistants, respiratory therapy students, and cardiac technology students.

This EKG book consists of 15 chapters designed to provide the user with a basic practical, yet comprehensive, approach to the skill of EKG interpretation. The strategy of this manuscript has centered on producing a useful guide to the understanding of abnormal heart rhythms, that is, dysrhythmias, for the health care provider in his or her provision of optimum patient care. In order to afford the instructor and the student the opportunity to work in a reasonable order through the technical information, the material has been presented in such a manner as to achieve understanding of each chapter prior to proceeding to the next chapter. The content is presented in short, succinct chapters in order to facilitate comprehension of each concept in a building-block format. Although the terms dysrhythmia and arrhythmia are synonymous, the term *dysrhythmia* is used throughout this book because I consider it to be the more correct and accurate description of the material presented.

In this revised fourth edition of the book, each chapter still contains a section of multiple-choice items to be used for self-assessment and review. The book includes expanded graphics, as well as rhythm strip examples with answers based on the five-step approach, review strips, key points to remember, chapter summary, and end-of-chapter questions to afford the student a comprehensive mastery of the material. Answers to review questions and review strips are provided in the appendices at the back of the book. Also included in this fourth edition of the book is a chapter dedicated to the assessment and management of the patient with cardiovascular emergencies.

An overview of major updates and additions to this revision may be helpful to you. These changes are summarized in the "What's New" list below.

WHAT'S NEW IN THE FOURTH EDITION

- Information has been updated to reflect current standards of care.
- Added and enhanced Chapter objectives and marginal glossary terms.
- Numerous review strip answers based on the five-step approach have been added.
- The feature Key Points to Remember has been enhanced and revised at the end of each chapter.
- End-of-Chapter Review Questions have been updated and revised.
- Instructor and student resources are available online at Brady's Resource Central Web site.

ResourceCentral

INSTRUCTOR RESOURCES

This Web site contains an array of instructor resources in one location. To access Resource Central, go to www.bradybooks.com and select myemskit/Resource Central. Click on the book cover for this title and follow registration/log-in instructions for Instructors. Your Brady sales representative can offer further assistance.

Once you are logged onto the site, you'll find the following teaching resources.

- PowerPoint Slides-updated and revised
- Lesson Plans
- Test Bank with more than 280 questions

STUDENT RESOURCES

This Web site provides chapter support materials and interactive resources in one location. To access Resource Central, follow directions on the Student Access Code Card provided with the text. If there is no card, go to www.bradybooks.com and select myemskit/Resource Central. Click on the book cover for this title and follow registration/Buy Access/log-in instructions for Students.

Once you are logged onto the site, you will find reinforcement exercises, enrichment activities, and links to additional references and support material.

It is my hope that you will find this book to be beneficial to your knowledge and comprehension of basic EKG interpretation. Your suggestions and comments are always welcome.

Brenda M. Beasley, RN, MS, EMT-Paramedic
Department Chair, Allied Health/EMS Program Director (Retired)
Calhoun Community College
E-mail address: bjm18@aol.com

Acknowledgments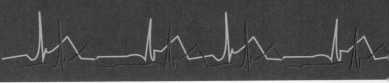

Just as the first three editions of this textbook were created from the challenges that I have experienced and the lessons I have learned throughout the past 35 years as a nurse, paramedic and an EMS educator, this revision was written to enhance the chapter content and, where appropriate, replace some of the content.

I have learned that the publication of textbooks involves many key people. I would like to acknowledge all the individuals who were instrumental, each in their own special way, in making the textbook revision possible. I also offer my sincere appreciation to the talented team members at Brady/Pearson Health Science who have led me through the revision process with expert advice, encouragement, and support. Thanks especially to Julie Alexander, Marlene Pratt, Sladjana Repic, Lois Berlowitz, Jonathan Cheung, Patrick Walsh, Patty Gutierrez, Debbie Ryan, and Brian Hoehl. My first editor at Brady, Judy Streger, has continued her support and encouragement throughout the years. Her belief in me has never waivered, and for that I am truly grateful.

My former EMS program faculty, both at Southern Union Community College and at Calhoun Community College (too many names to mention here, but they know who they are!), have all been my strength and inspiration to strive for excellence in EMS education. The reviewers of this book, whose names follow, offered important perspective. Their comments and suggestions have been very valuable.

Mike West has continued to be my champion and has worked closely with me throughout this revision process. His encouragement and constancy were very critical to me, and I wish to thank him for the long hours he spent working with me on this revision, as well as for his valuable assistance in gathering and incorporating the new changes and additions to the review questions and EKG strips.

The memory of my mother and my father, who taught my sisters and me to believe first in God, then in our family, and ultimately in ourselves; they always provided me with unconditional love, acceptance, and a solid foundation upon which to build a life.

It is my belief that every novice author is, at some point, inspired by other authors, and colleagues who transition to mentors, role models, and precious friends. In my particular case, there were many. I especially appreciate the support and friendship of the following EMS colleagues: Walt Stoy, Joe Mistovich, Greg Margolis, Jeff Lindsey, Dwayne Clayden, Bryan Bledsoe, Baxter Larmon, and Dan Limmer.

And last, but not least, I gratefully acknowledge my family, friends, and colleagues, for they are the true "contributors" to this product. Their contributions include love, patience, support, encouragement, and acceptance of my erratic schedule during the text revision.

REVIEWERS

I wish to thank the following reviewers for providing invaluable feedback and suggestions during the revision of this text:

James "Bud" Adams, AAS, NREMT-P
Instructor of Emergency Medicine College of Southern Nevada Las Vegas, NV

John L Beckman, AA, BS, FF/EMT-P
EMS Instructor Addison Fire Protection District Addison, IL

Deborah K. Drummonds, RN, MN, CCRN, CEN
Assistant Professor School of Nursing and Health Sciences Abraham Baldwin Agricultural College Tifton, GA

Fidel O. Garcia, EMT-P
President/Owner Professional EMS Education,
LLC Grand Junction, CO

Stephanie Morrison, RN, BSN
ACLS Instructor Thomas Hospital Fairhope, AL

David Pierce, BA, NREMT-P
EMS Faculty Century College White Bear Lake, MN

Shari Turner, M.Ed., EMT-P
Palm Beach Gardens, FL

Randy Williams, NREMT-P
EMS Programs Coordinator Bainbridge College
Bainbridge, GA

I also wish to thank the following professionals who reviewed earlier editions of *Understanding EKGs: A Practical Approach*:

John L. Beckman, AA, BS, FF/EMT-P Instructor
Affiliated with Addison Fire Protection District
Fire Science Instructor, Technology Center of
DuPage Addison, IL

Mark Branon, BS, NREMT-P
EMS Program Director Calhoun Community
College Decatur, AL

Art Breault, RN, EMT-Paramedic
Niskayuna Fire District No. 1 Albany Medical
Center Hospital—Department of Emergency
Medicine Albany, NY

Benjamin J. Camp, MD, FACEP
Chief of Staff Tanner Health System Emergency
Services Carrollton, GA

Greg Charma, AAS, NREMT-P
Paramedic/Assistant EMS Training Director
Tucson Fire Department Pima Community
College Tucson, AZ

Marilyn Ermish, NREMT-P
American Medical Response Cheyenne, WY

Jason Ferguson, BPA, NREMT-P
EMS Programs Head Central Virginia Community
College Lynchburg, VA

Scott Garrett
Director of Education Upstate EMS Council
Greenville, SC

Craig H. Jacobus, D.C.; NREMT-P; EMSI
Links 4 Life Metro Community College ALS
Affiliates Lincoln Medical Education Partnership
(LMEP) Schuyler, NE

Scott Jones
Director—Paramedic Academy Victor Valley
College Victorville, CA

Maryla Kathryn Lee, RN, BSN, MSN
Calhoun Community College Decatur, AL

Jeff McDonald
Coordinator, Emergency Medical Services
Program Tarrant Count College—Northeast
Campus Hurst, TX

Mike McEvoy, PhD, EMT-P, RN, CCRN
Saratoga County EMS Coordinator Clinical
Associate Professor in Critical Care Medicine
Albany Medical College Waterford, NY

Steve McGraw
Assistant Professor The George Washington
University School of Medicine and Health
Sciences Washington, DC

Regina Pearson, EMT-P
Clinical Coordinator/Instructor, Emergency
Medical Technology Jackson State Community
College Jackson, TN

Jonathan Smith, NREMT-P
Lead Paramedic Instructor Chattahoochee
Technical College Acworth, GA

Thomas Y. Smith, Sr.
Fire Science/EMS Program Director West Georgia
Technical College LaGrange, GA

Scott R. Snyder, BS, NREMT-P.
Primary EMT Instructor San Francisco Paramedic
Association San Francisco, CA

Andrew E. Spain
Assistant Manager, Emergency Services
University of Missouri Health Care EMS
Education Columbia, MO

Carl Voskamp, LP
Coordinator of EMS and Firefighting Programs
The Victoria College Victoria, TX

Jim Williams, CCEMT-P, NREMT-P
Training Officer, Medical Center EMS Bowling
Green, KY

About the Author

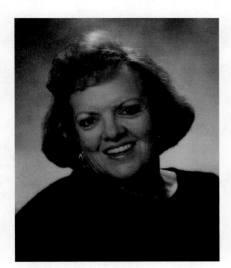

Brenda Messer Beasley is a paramedic and a registered nurse. She earned her bachelor's and master's degree, as well as additional postgraduate studies, from the University of Alabama and from Lorenz University, respectively. Following graduation from nursing school at the University of Alabama, Ms. Beasley was employed as a nurse in the Emergency Department of University Hospital in Birmingham. She remained in emergency nursing for the next 10 years, with a 2-year hiatus when she became certified as a critical care neurosurgical nurse and worked in an NICU at Carraway Medical Center.

Ms. Beasley was working as an ER nurse in 1978 when she was asked to teach a basic EMT course. With a great deal of reticence yet strong encouragement from the chief of staff at the local hospital, she concurred. She immediately developed a passion for quality EMS education, and the rest, as they say, is history. For the next 30 years, she served as an EMS educator in the state of Alabama, and in 2001 was named Department Chair of Allied Health at Calhoun Community College in Decatur, Alabama. She held that position until her retirement in 2007.

Ms. Beasley was an affiliate faculty member of the American Heart Association's Emergency Cardiac Care Program for 25 years. Other professional activities include BTLS affiliate faculty and board of directors of the National Association of EMS Educators, and she serves on the medical advisory boards of Action Training Systems and Southern Ambulance Transport.

In 1999, Ms. Beasley published her first book on EKG interpretation and has subsequently authored other texts for Brady/Pearson Health Science. She resides in Wedowee, Alabama, (with her beloved pet, Kitty Boo) where she serves as vice chair of the local hospital board. Ms. Beasley is actively involved in the First United Methodist Church of Wedowee and currently serves as the Governance Committee Chair for the National Association of EMS Educators.

PAC?—

PVC? wid aVs

PJC?—Normal aVs

JUCTION? inverted P wave or no P wave.

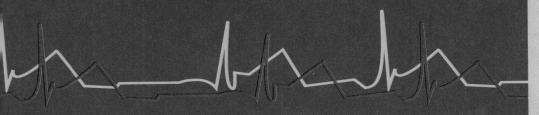

The Anatomy of the Heart: Structure

INTRODUCTION

A thorough understanding of the structure of the heart provides the student with a foundation upon which to build the knowledge of basic dysrhythmia interpretation. Therefore, the focus of this chapter will be to provide you, the student, with a simple yet comprehensive understanding of cardiac anatomy. After you have mastered the knowledge of basic cardiac anatomy (structure), you will be prepared to move to Chapter 2, which addresses the basic physiology (function) of the heart.

ANATOMY OF THE HEART

First you must realize that the heart is a muscle. Although we don't think of exercising our heart muscle when we go to the gym, the fact is that your heart muscle (myocardium) is constantly in the "exercise mode." At times of rest, the exercise is more sedate. Think, however, of the vigor with which your heart muscle must exercise when you walk (or run) up six flights of stairs! Now as you feel your heart pumping, you can easily understand that your heart muscle is indeed exercising.

We often hear the heart referred to as a "two-sided pump," and this analogy works well in our understanding of the basics of cardiac anatomy. Indeed, we can visualize this pump as having a right side and a left side. On each side of the pump, there is an upper chamber of the heart, which is referred to as the **atrium** (atria, plural), and a lower chamber of the heart known as the **ventricle**. In all, there are four hollow chambers in the normal heart. Again, the two upper chambers of the heart are called atria; the two lower chambers are called ventricles.

Separating the upper chambers is the interatrial septum. The lower, inferior chambers are separated by the interventricular septum. (See ■ **Figure 1–1**.) Externally, the atrioventricular groove, known as the **coronary sulcus**, surrounds the outside of the heart and divides the atria from the ventricles. The anterior and posterior interventricular grooves separate the ventricles externally. The muscle fibers of the ventricles are continuous, as are the atrial muscle fibers.

The two upper chambers of the heart are located at the base, or top, of the heart; the lower chambers are located at the bottom, or apex, of the heart. The upper chambers of the heart are thin walled and receive blood as it returns to the heart. The lower chambers of the heart have thicker walls and pump blood away from the heart, throughout the systemic circulation and to the myocardium.

atrium upper chamber of the heart

ventricle lower chamber of the heart

coronary sulcus the atrioventricular groove that surrounds the outside of the heart and divides the atria from the ventricles

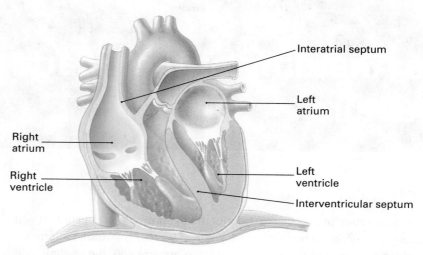

FIGURE 1–1. The chambers of the heart

LOCATION, SIZE, AND SHAPE OF THE HEART

It is important for you to learn and understand the location of the heart in that the effectiveness of one of our most basic and most important skills—CPR—depends upon a reasonable knowledge of this position. In addition, the proper placement of electrodes to record an electrocardiogram, which is discussed in Chapter 5, depends upon the proper understanding of the location of the heart.

The central section of the thorax (chest cavity) is called the **mediastinum**. It is in this area that the heart and its large vessels are housed, lying in front of the spinal column, behind the sternum, and between the lungs. (See ■ **Figure 1–2**.) Also located in the mediastinum are the trachea, esophagus, thymus, lymph nodes, and other structures and tissues.

mediastinum the central section of the thorax (chest cavity)

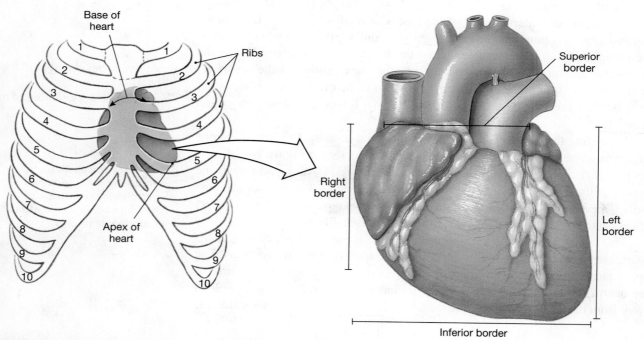

FIGURE 1–2. Position and orientation of the heart within the mediastinum

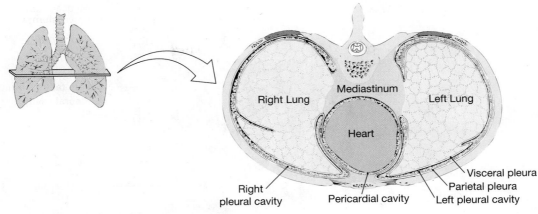

FIGURE 1–3. Anatomical relationships in the thoracic cavity

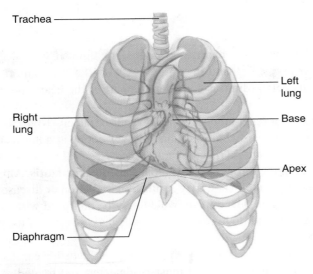

FIGURE 1–4. Location of the heart within the chest

When thinking of the heart muscle in terms of its mass, one should realize that two-thirds of the heart muscle lies to the left of the midline. The apex of the heart lies just above the diaphragm. The base of the heart lies at approximately the level of the third rib. (See ■ Figures 1–2 and 1–4.)

The exact size of the heart varies somewhat among individuals, but on average it is approximately 5 inches (in.), or 12 centimeters (cm), in length and 3 in., or 7.5 cm, wide. The shape of the heart is somewhat conelike. It is appropriate to visualize the heart as approximately the size of the owner's closed fist. (See ■ Figure 1–3.)

LAYERS OF THE HEART

Pericardium

Surrounding the heart is a closed, two-layered sac referred to as the **pericardium**, or pericardial sac. In direct contact with the pleura is the outer layer or parietal pericardium. (See ■ Figure 1–5.) This layer consists of tough, inelastic fibrous connective tissue and serves

pericardium closed, two-layered sac that surrounds the heart

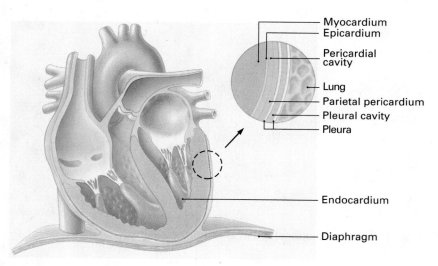

FIGURE 1–5. Layers of the heart

to prevent overdistention of the heart. The thin, serous inner layer of the pericardium is called the visceral pericardium and is contiguous with the epicardium, which surrounds the heart. The serous pericardium is considered a part of the heart and is continuous with the epicardium.

A space filled with a scant amount of fluid (approximately 10 to 50 cubic centimeters [cc]) separates the two pericardial layers. This fluid, by acting as a lubricant, helps to reduce friction as the heart moves within the pericardial sac.

pericarditis an inflammation of the serous pericardium

An inflammation of the serous pericardium is called **pericarditis**. Although the cause of this disease is frequently unknown, it may result from infection or disease of the connective tissue. Pericarditis can cause severe pain, which may be confused with or mistaken for the pain of a myocardial infarction. This can make physical assessment of the patient a real challenge for the clinician.

An excess accumulation of fluid in the pericardial sac is called cardiac tamponade. This condition is an extreme emergency and must be detected and treated expeditiously. (See Chapter 13 for discussion.)

The heart wall

epicardium the smooth outer surface of the heart

myocardium the thick middle layer of the heart composed primarily of cardiac muscle cells and responsible for the heart's ability to contract

endocardium the innermost layer of the heart; composed of thin connective tissue

Three primary layers of tissue comprise the heart wall. (See Figure 1–5.) This specialized cardiac muscle tissue is unique to the heart. The **epicardium** accounts for the smooth outer surface of the heart. The main coronary arteries are located on the surface of the epicardium. The thick middle layer of the heart is called the **myocardium** and is the thickest of the three layers of the heart wall. The myocardium is composed primarily of cardiac muscle cells and is responsible for the heart's ability to contract. The innermost layer, the **endocardium**, is composed of endothelial tissue. This area requires a constant and uninterrupted supply of oxygen and is subject to ischemia (decreased supply of oxygenated blood). This smooth inner surface of the heart and heart valves serves to allow blood to flow more easily throughout the heart.

VALVES OF THE HEART

The four valves of the heart allow blood to flow in only one direction. (See ■ **Figure 1–6**.) There are two sets of valves, the atrioventricular valves and the semilunar valves.

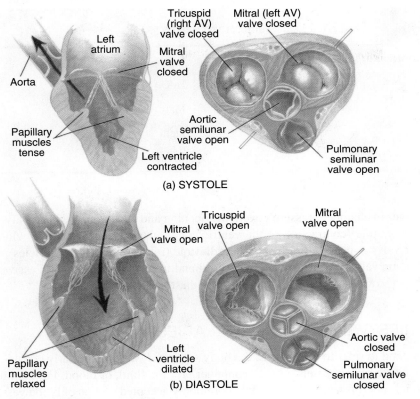

Tricuspid (right AV) valve closed
Mitral (left AV) valve closed
Left atrium
Mitral valve closed
Aorta
Papillary muscles tense
Aortic semilunar valve open
Left ventricle contracted
Pulmonary semilunar valve open

(a) SYSTOLE

Tricuspid valve open
Mitral valve open
Mitral valve open
Aortic valve closed
Papillary muscles relaxed
Left ventricle dilated
Pulmonary semilunar valve closed

(b) DIASTOLE

FIGURE 1–6. Valves of the heart

Atrioventricular valves

As the term indicates, the atrioventricular valves are located between the atria and the ventricles. These valves allow blood to flow from the atria into the ventricles. They are also effective in preventing the blood from flowing backward from the ventricles into the atria. The **tricuspid valve** is named for its three cusps and is located between the right atrium and the right ventricle.

Free edges of each of the three cusps extend into the ventricles, where they attach to the chordae tendineae. **Chordae tendineae** are fine chords of dense connective tissue that attach to papillary muscles in the wall of the ventricles. Chordae tendineae and papillary muscles (see Figure 1–6) work in concert to prevent the cusps from fluttering back into the atrium and disrupting blood flow through the heart.

The **mitral (or bicuspid) valve** (see Figure 1–6) is similar in structure to the tricuspid valve, but has only two cusps. The mitral valve is located between the left atrium and the left ventricle.

The mnemonic in ■ **Table 1–1** has proved helpful in recalling the location of the atrioventricular valves.

Semilunar valves

Much as the atrioventricular valves prevent backflow of blood into the atria, the **semilunar valves** serve to prevent the backflow of blood into the ventricles. Each semilunar valve contains three semilunar (or moon-shaped) cusps. The semilunar valves are the pulmonic and aortic valves. The semilunar valve located between the right ventricle and the pulmonary artery is called the **pulmonic valve**. The semilunar valve located between the left ventricle and the trunk of the aorta is called the **aortic valve** (Figure 1–6).

tricuspid valve named for its three cusps; located between the right atrium and the right ventricle

chordae tendineae fine chords of dense connective tissue that attach to papillary muscles in the wall of the ventricles

mitral (or bicuspid) valve similar in structure to the tricuspid valve but with only two cusps and is located between the left atrium and the left ventricle

semilunar valves serve to prevent the backflow of blood into the ventricles, each valve containing three semilunar (or moon-shaped) cusps

pulmonic valve the semilunar valve located between the right ventricle and the pulmonary artery

aortic valve the semilunar valve located between the left ventricle and the trunk of the aorta

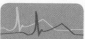

TABLE 1–1 Mnemonic: Heart valves

Atrioventricular Valves	
L	Left
M	Mitral
R	Right
T	Tricuspid

Changes in chamber pressure govern the opening and closing of the heart valves. During ventricular systole (contraction of the ventricles), the atrioventricular valves close and the semilunar valves open. During ventricular diastole (relaxation of the ventricles), the aortic and pulmonic valves are closed and the mitral and tricuspid valves open. Passive filling of the coronary arteries occurs during ventricular diastole.

ARTERIES, VEINS, AND CAPILLARIES

Since we tend to refer to the heart as the body's "pump," we can similarly consider the vasculature, or the blood vessels, as the "container" for the fluid, or blood. For the purposes of this text, it is appropriate to discuss three commonly accepted groups of blood vessels: arteries, veins, and capillaries. (See ■ **Figure 1–7**.)

Arteries

arteries thick walled and muscular blood vessels that function under high pressure to convey blood from the heart out to the rest of the body

Arteries, by virtue of their primary function, are relatively thick walled and muscular. These blood vessels function under high pressure in order to convey blood from the heart out to the rest of the body. The prefix *a* can mean away from, and so it is helpful to remember that the word artery also begins with the letter *a*; thus arteries carry blood away from the heart. Larger arterial blood vessels are called arteries, and these vessels branch off into smaller blood vessels known as arterioles. Arteries carry oxygenated blood, with the exception of the pulmonary and umbilical arteries.

Arteries also operate in the regulation of blood pressure through functional changes in peripheral vascular resistance. Arterial walls consist of three distinct layers: the intima, media, and adventitia. (See ■ **Table 1–2** and ■ **Figure 1–8**.) These layers are also called tunics (coats or coverings). The tunica intima is the innermost layer and consists of endothelium and an inner elastic membrane. This inner elastic membrane separates the intimal layer from the next layer, the tunica media. The tunica media is the middle layer and consists of smooth muscle cells. In this middle layer, the blood flow through the vessel is regulated by constriction or dilation. Vasoconstriction, a decrease in the diameter of the blood vessel, produces a decrease in blood flow. In contrast, vasodilation, an increase in the diameter of the blood vessel, produces an increase in blood flow. The tunica adventitia, or outermost layer, is composed of various connective tissues.

Coronary arteries and the coronary sinus

The primary structures of importance in this section are the coronary arteries and the coronary sinus. (See ■ **Figure 1–9**.)

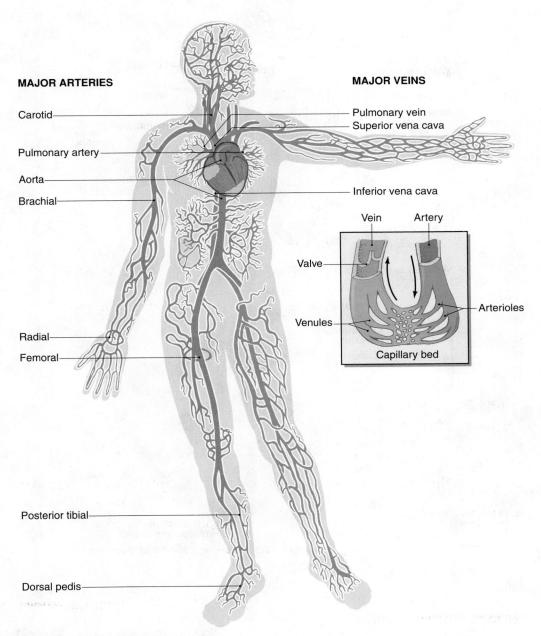

MAJOR ARTERIES

Carotid

Pulmonary artery

Aorta

Brachial

Radial

Femoral

Posterior tibial

Dorsal pedis

MAJOR VEINS

Pulmonary vein
Superior vena cava

Inferior vena cava

Vein   Artery

Valve

Venules

Arterioles

Capillary bed

FIGURE 1–7. Circulatory system

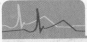 **TABLE 1–2 Arterial Wall Layers**

Name	Layer	Tissue Type
Tunica intima	Innermost	Connective and elastic
Tunica media	Middle	Smooth muscle, elastic, and collagen
Tunica adventitia	Outermost	Connective

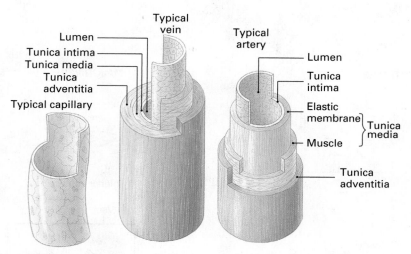

FIGURE 1–8. Arterial wall layers

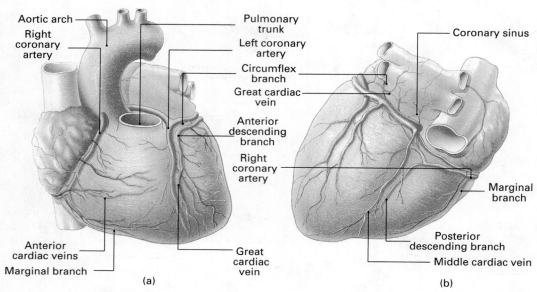

FIGURE 1–9. Coronary circulation

Two Main Coronary Arteries

coronary arteries
the two main arteries that arise from the trunk of the aorta and function to carry oxygenated blood throughout the myocardium

coronary circulation
the process by which oxygenated blood is distributed throughout the heart muscle

Two main **coronary arteries**, the right and left, arise from the trunk of the aorta and function to carry oxygenated blood throughout the myocardium. These arteries branch off into smaller vessels to supply the heart with oxygenated blood. Because the left side of the heart is more muscular than the right side, the left coronary artery branches are more muscular than the right coronary artery branches. Oxygenated blood is distributed throughout the heart muscle through the process known as **coronary circulation**.

As the left coronary artery leaves the aorta, it immediately divides into the left anterior descending artery and the circumflex artery. The anterior descending artery is the major branch of the left coronary artery and supplies blood to most of the anterior part of the heart. A marginal branch of the left coronary artery supplies blood to the lateral wall of the left ventricle. The circumflex branch of the left coronary artery extends around to the posterior side of the heart, and its branches supply blood to much of the posterior wall of the heart. Each of these divisions has numerous branches that form a network of blood vessels, which in turn serve to provide oxygenation of designated portions of the myocardium.

The right coronary artery extends from the aorta around to the posterior portion of the heart. Branches of the right coronary artery supply blood to the lateral wall of the right ventricle. A branch of the right coronary artery called the posterior interventricular artery or posterior descending artery lies in the posterior interventricular region and supplies blood to the posterior and inferior part of the heart's left ventricle. The right coronary artery branches also supply oxygen-rich blood to a portion of the electrical conduction system.

Coronary Sinus

The **coronary sinus** (also referred to as the "Great Cardiac Vein") is a short trunk that serves to receive deoxygenated blood from the veins of the myocardium. This trunk empties into the right atrium. (See Figure 1–9.)

Veins

Veins are defined as blood vessels that carry blood back to the heart. Veins branch off into smaller vessels known as **venules**. With the exception of venules, veins are structurally similar to arteries in that they also have three layers. Unlike arteries, however, veins operate under low pressure, are relatively thin walled, and contain one-way valves. With the exception of the pulmonary vein, the veins convey deoxygenated blood.

The larger veins of the body ultimately empty into the two largest veins, the **superior vena cava** and the **inferior vena cava**, which empty deoxygenated blood into the heart's right atrium. The superior vena cava drains blood from the head and neck. The inferior vena cava collects blood from the rest of the body. (See Figure 1–7.)

Capillaries

Capillaries are tiny blood vessels whose walls are the thinnest of all blood vessels. There are more capillaries in the human body than any other blood vessel. In fact, capillaries are so tiny that red blood cells must "march through" in single file. From the arterioles, blood flows into the capillaries, where the vast majority of gas exchange occurs.

In summary, arterioles transport oxygenated blood into the capillaries. Capillaries allow for the exchange of oxygen, nutrients, and waste products between the blood and body tissues and are viewed as "connectors" between arteries and veins. The smallest of the veins, the venules, then receive the deoxygenated blood, which travels back to the heart via the venous system. To get a clearer picture of blood flow through the various vessels, please refer to ■ **Figure 1–10**.

This chapter would not be complete without a brief discussion of the circulatory system. **Circulation** refers to movement through a course (the body) that leads back to the initial point (the heart). Two major components comprise the circulatory system, the pulmonary circulation and the systemic circulation.

PULMONARY CIRCULATION

A rudimentary way to remember pulmonary circulation is to recall that it is the blood flow between the heart and lungs. When blood leaves the heart through the right ventricle and travels into the pulmonary artery to the lungs and back through the pulmonary veins to the left atrium, the cycle is known as **pulmonary circulation**. The importance of this component of the circulatory system cannot be overemphasized. The critical concept of **tissue perfusion** is based on adequate gas exchange within the alveolar capillary membranes in the lungs.

---

coronary sinus (also referred to as the "Great Cardiac Vein") a short trunk that serves to receive deoxygenated blood from the veins of the myocardium

veins blood vessels that carry blood back to the heart, operate under low pressure, and are relatively thin walled

superior vena cava drains blood from the head and neck

inferior vena cava collects blood from the rest of the body

capillaries tiny blood vessels that allow for the exchange of oxygen, nutrients, and waste products between the blood and body tissues; "connectors" between arteries and veins

circulation movement through a course (the body) that leads back to the initial point (the heart)

pulmonary circulation when blood leaves the heart through the right ventricle and travels into the **pulmonary artery** to the lungs and back through the pulmonary veins to the left atrium

tissue perfusion refers to gas exchange within the alveolar capillary membranes in the lungs.

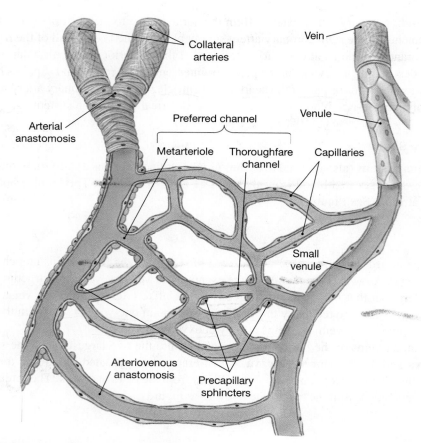

FIGURE 1–10. Organization of capillary bed

systemic circulation
the circulation of blood as it leaves the left ventricle and travels through the arteries, capillaries, and veins of the entire body system and back to the primary receptacle of the heart (the right atrium)

SYSTEMIC CIRCULATION

Systemic circulation consists of the circulation of blood as it leaves the left ventricle and travels through the arteries, capillaries, and veins of the entire body system and back to the primary receptacle of the heart (the right atrium). Maintenance of each tissue type in the body is ensured by the work of the systemic and pulmonary circulations, collectively.

CHAPTER 1

 SUMMARY

Your understanding of the anatomy of the heart and blood vessels will become increasingly important as you move from chapter to chapter in this book. It is not possible to have a thorough understanding of dysrhythmias and their causes unless you also have an excellent grasp of cardiovascular anatomy.

KEY POINTS TO REMEMBER

1. The heart is located in the mediastinum and lies in front of the spinal column behind the sternum and between the lungs.

2. The apex (bottom) of the heart lies just above the diaphragm; the base of the heart lies at approximately the level of the third rib.

3. It is appropriate to visualize the heart as approximately the size of the owner's closed fist.

4. There are a total of four hollow chambers in the normal heart on each side of the heart. There is an upper chamber, which is referred to as the atrium (atria, plural) and a lower chamber known as the ventricle.

5. Surrounding the heart is a closed, two-layered sac referred to as the pericardium, which is also known as the pericardial sac.

6. The epicardium accounts for the smooth outer surface of the heart.

7. The thick, middle layer of the heart is the myocardium and is the thickest of the three layers of the heart wall.

8. The innermost layer, the endocardium, is composed of thin connective tissue.

9. The atrioventricular valves are located between the atria and the ventricles and allow blood to flow from the atria into the ventricles.

10. The semilunar valves serve to prevent the backflow of blood into the ventricles; contain three semilunar (or moon-shaped) cusps. They are the pulmonic and aortic valves.

11. Arteries are relatively thick walled and muscular in structure and function under high pressure.

12. Veins are blood vessels that carry blood back to the heart and operate under low pressure.

13. Capillaries are tiny blood vessels (whose walls are the thinnest of all blood vessels); they allow for the exchange of oxygen, nutrients, and waste products.

REVIEW QUESTIONS

1. The fibrous sac covering of the heart, which is in contact with the pleura, is the:
   a. Epicardium
   b. Myocardium
   c. Pericardium
   d. Endocardium

2. The lower chamber of the heart, with the thickest myocardium, is the:
   a. Right
   b. Left

3. The pulmonic and aortic valves are open during:
   a. Systole
   b. Diastole

4. The large blood vessel that returns unoxygenated blood from the head and neck to the right atrium is called the:
   a. Jugular vein
   b. Carotid artery
   c. Superior vena cava
   d. Inferior vena cava

5. The right coronary artery branches supply oxygen-rich blood to a portion of the:
   a. Electrical conduction system
   b. Left circumflex arteries
   c. Sympathetic nervous system
   d. Coronary sinus

6. The most numerous blood vessels in the body are the:
   a. Arteries
   b. Capillaries
   c. Venules
   d. Veins

7. Blood flow between the heart and lungs is _____ circulation.
   a. Systemic
   b. Venous
   c. Myocardial
   d. Pulmonary

8. These blood vessels function under high pressure in order to convey blood from the heart out to the rest of the body:
   a. Venules
   b. Veins
   c. Arteries
   d. Capillaries

9. An inflammation of the serous pericardium is called:
   a. Myocarditis
   b. Pericarditis
   c. Pulmonitis
   d. Tendonitis

10. The smooth outer surface of the heart is called the:
    a. Pericardium   c. Epicardium
    b. Endocardium   d. Myocardium

11. The _____ valve is named for its three cusps and is located between the right atrium and the right ventricle.
    a. Bicuspid   c. Aortic
    b. Tricuspid   d. Pulmonic

12. Chordae tendineae and papillary muscles work in concert to prevent the cusps from fluttering back into the:
    a. Atrium   c. Aorta
    b. Ventricle   d. Vena cava

13. The right and left coronary arteries arise from the:
    a. Left ventricle   c. Coronary sinus
    b. Right atrium   d. Trunk of the aorta

14. The central section of the thorax (chest cavity) is called the:
    a. Costal margin   c. Diaphragm
    b. Mediastinum   d. Xiphoid

15. The apex of the heart lies just above the:
    a. Intercostal space c. Diaphragm
    b. Mediastinum   d. Xiphoid

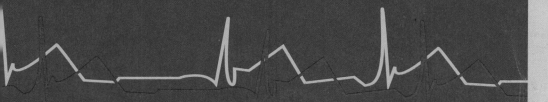

Cardiovascular Physiology: Function

2

Objectives

Upon completion of this chapter, the student will be able to:

- Explain the sequence of blood flow through the heart
- Describe the cardiac cycle, including
  a. Definition
  b. Systole
  c. Diastole
- Discuss the term stroke volume
- Explain cardiac output
- Discuss preload and afterload
- Discuss Starling's Law
- Describe the autonomic nervous system, including the:
  - Sympathetic nervous system, and the
  - Parasympathetic nervous system

INTRODUCTION

Now that we have addressed the structure of the heart, we will discuss the basic function, or physiology, of the cardiovascular system. We will build on the foundation provided in Chapters 1 and 2 as we sequentially discuss each chapter in order to gain a thorough knowledge of interpreting basic dysrhythmias. The focus of this chapter is to provide you, the student, with an uncomplicated yet inclusive look at the basics of cardiac physiology. After you have mastered the knowledge of basic cardiac physiology, or function, you will be prepared to move on to Chapter 3, which addresses the basic electrophysiology of the heart.

NOTE: Now is the perfect time to look back at the review questions from Chapter 1. Then proceed through the objectives and contents of this chapter.

BLOOD FLOW THROUGH THE HEART

The path of blood flow through the heart (■ **Figure 2–1**) is our first consideration in acquiring knowledge of the physiology of circulation. Imagine, if you will, that the right atrium is a receptacle functioning in part to receive deoxygenated blood from the head, neck, and trunk. In order to simplify the route of circulation, the learner may choose to divide this concept into three components.

The first component would consist of blood flow through the right atrium, which proceeds as follows. Deoxygenated blood flows from the inferior and superior vena cavae into the:

Right atrium	Through the tricuspid valve	Into the right Ventricle	Through the pulmonic valve

The second component of blood flow through the pulmonary circulation continues when the blood travels from the pulmonic valve into the:

Pulmonary arteries	Into the lungs	Through the pulmonary alveolar-capillary network	Into the Pulmonary Veins

The third and final component of blood flow through the pulmonary circulation continues when the blood travels from the pulmonary veins into the:

Left atrium	Through the mitral valve	Into the left ventricle	Through the aortic valve and out to the rest of the body

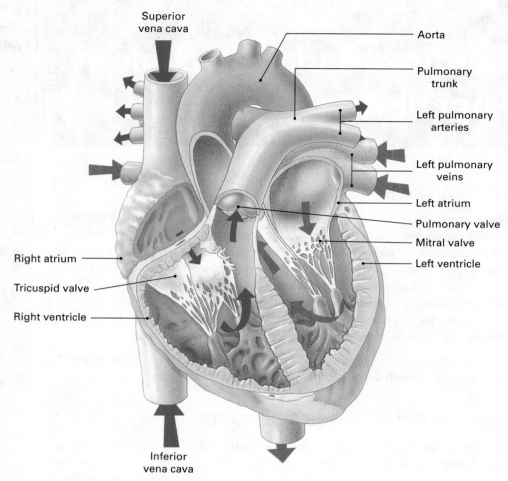

FIGURE 2–1. Blood flow through the heart

It should be noted that the freshly oxygenated blood, traveling through the aortic valve, also enters the coronary arteries during diastole, when the aortic valve closes, to accomplish myocardial oxygenation. The vital function of gas exchange occurs in the seconds or middle component of pulmonary circulation when carbon dioxide is exchanged for oxygen in the pulmonary alveolar-capillary network.

CARDIAC CYCLE

The heart functions as a unit in that both atria contract simultaneously, and then both ventricles contract. (See ■ **Figure 2–2**.) When the atria contract, the ventricles are filled to their limit. Blood is ejected into the pulmonary and systemic circulations when simultaneous contraction of the ventricles occurs. At the time of ventricular contraction, the mitral and tricuspid valves are closed by the pressure of the contraction, whereas the pulmonic and aortic valves are opened. The **cardiac cycle** represents the actual time sequence between ventricular contraction and ventricular relaxation.

Systole, also referred to as **ventricular systole**, is consistent with the simultaneous contraction of the ventricles, whereas **diastole** is synonymous with ventricular relaxation. The ventricles fill passively with approximately 70 percent of the blood that has collected in the atria during ventricular diastole. Then the active contraction of the atria propels the remaining 30 percent of the blood into the ventricles. Atrial contraction has only a minimal role in filling;

cardiac cycle
the actual time sequence between ventricular contraction and ventricular relaxation

systole, or ventricular systole
is consistent with the simultaneous contraction of the ventricles

diastole is synonymous with ventricular relaxation

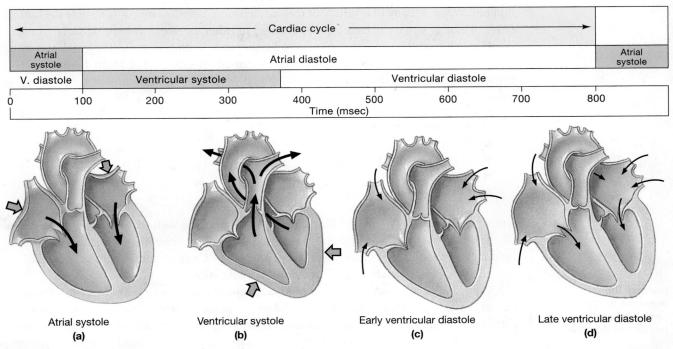

FIGURE 2–2. Cardiac cycle

consequently, even if the atria do not contract effectively, ventricular filling still ensues. During periods of ventricular relaxation, cardiac filling and coronary perfusion occur passively.

One cardiac cycle occurs every 0.8 seconds. Systole lasts about 0.28 seconds. Diastole lasts about 0.52 seconds. Therefore, the period of diastole is substantially longer than the period of systole. The amount of blood pumped out of the ventricle with each cardiac cycle can be measured most often by an ultrasound of the heart (echocardiograph). This measurement is referred to as ejection fraction (EF), with a normal value of 55 to 70 percent. An EF of less than 40 percent is indicative of heart failure and less than 35 percent may indicate life-threatening dysrhythmias and lead to sudden cardiac death.

STROKE VOLUME

Stroke volume may be defined as the volume of blood pumped out of one ventricle of the heart in a single beat or contraction. Stroke volume is estimated at approximately 70 cubic centimeters (cc) or milliliters (ml) per beat. The number of contractions, or beats per minute (BPM), is known as the **heart rate**. The normal adult heart rate is 60 to 100 BPM.

CARDIAC OUTPUT

Cardiac output is the amount of blood pumped by the left ventricle in 1 minute (min). The output of the right ventricle is normally equal to the left because these two chambers contract simultaneously.

By remembering the following formula, we can determine the cardiac output:

Cardiac output (CO) =	Stroke volume (SV) × Heart rate (HR)

Consequently, if a patient has a heart rate of 80 BPM and a stroke volume of 70 cc per beat, the resulting cardiac output will be approximately 5600 cc per minute (or 5.6 liters [L] per

stroke volume the volume of blood pumped out of one ventricle of the heart in a single beat or contraction

heart rate the number of contractions, or beats, per minute of the heart

cardiac output the amount of blood pumped by the left ventricle in 1 min

minute). When, for any of a variety of reasons, a patient's cardiac output is outside the normal range, the heart will try to balance it by changes in either the stroke volume or the heart rate.

Cardiac output varies from person to person and depends upon activity and metabolic demands. Inadequate cardiac output may be caused by Congestive Heart Failure (CHF), myocardial infarction (MI), or shock and may be indicated by any combination of the following signs and symptoms:

- Shortness of breath
- Dizziness
- Decreased blood pressure
- Chest pains
- Cool and clammy skin

Note that patients may exhibit other signs and symptoms as well. If your patient complains of chest pain and begins to exhibit any of the signs and symptoms of inadequate cardiac output, you should immediately contact a physician. Cardiac output can be increased by exercise, increased metabolic rate, and cardiac medications.

Commonly called end-diastolic pressure, **preload** is the pressure in the ventricles at the end of diastole. Preload is directly affected by the exact volume of blood that returns to the right atrium and may be decreased or increased, based on the returning volume. **Afterload** is the resistance against which the heart must pump. This pressure also affects stroke volume and cardiac output.

When the volume of blood in the ventricles is increased, this causes stretching of the ventricular myocardial fibers and, consequently, a more forceful contraction. This concept is known as **Starling's Law of the heart**. This law of physiology basically states that the more the myocardial fibers are stretched, up to a certain point, the more forceful the subsequent contraction will be. Thus we can assume that if the volume of blood filling the ventricle increases significantly, so will the force of the cardiac contraction. This may be thought of as analogous to the stretching of a rubber band; thus we have the "rubber band theory": The farther you stretch a rubber band, the harder it snaps back to its original size. As a result, as the heart beats faster, the less volume of blood it can pump out, thus decreasing efficiency.

The amount of opposition to blood flow offered by the arterioles is known as **peripheral vascular resistance (PVR)** or systemic vascular resistance (SVR). A patient's blood pressure may increase or decrease if the cardiac output changes significantly and the peripheral vascular resistance remains uniform. Vasoconstriction and vasodilation determine peripheral vascular resistance. Blood pressure is subject to change if the cardiac output or peripheral vascular resistance changes.

Therefore, it may be helpful to remember the following formula:

Blood pressure (BP) =	Cardiac output (CO) × Peripheral vascular resistance (PVR)

AUTONOMIC NERVOUS SYSTEM

When we consider all the pathophysiological processes that are required in order to maintain homeostasis, or equilibrium, in the internal environment of our bodies, we quickly realize that we are fortunate to possess a built-in control center. This control center is known as the **autonomic nervous system (ANS)**.

The autonomic nervous system regulates functions of the body that are involuntary, or not under conscious control. In other words, we do not have to consciously think about our every heartbeat or about regulating our blood pressure. Heart rate and blood pressure are regulated by this component of the nervous system. (See ■ **Figure 2–3**.)

preload the pressure in the ventricles at the end of diastole

afterload the resistance against which the heart must pump

Starling's Law of the heart the more the myocardial fibers are stretched, up to a certain point, the more forceful the subsequent contraction will be

peripheral vascular resistance (PVR) the amount of opposition to blood flow offered by the arterioles

autonomic nervous system (ANS) regulates functions of the body that are involuntary, or not under conscious control

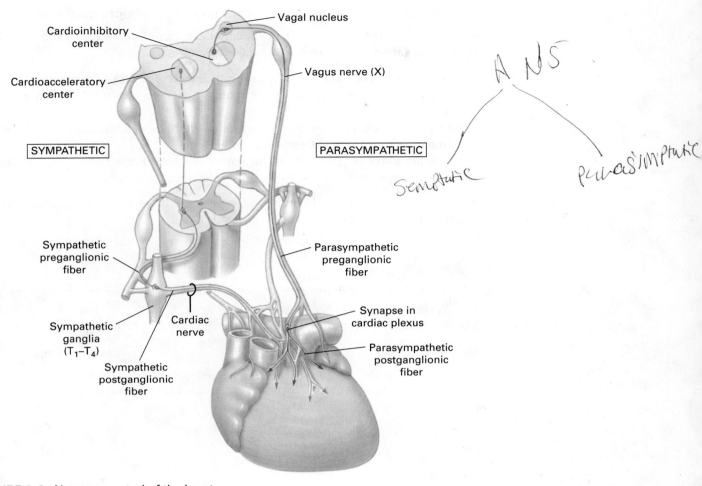

FIGURE 2–3. Nervous control of the heart

There are two major divisions of the ANS: the sympathetic nervous system and the parasympathetic nervous system. The majority of organs in the body are innervated by both systems. It is important to note that blood vessels are innervated only by the sympathetic nervous system. The **sympathetic nervous system** is responsible for preparation of the body for physical activity (fight or flight). The **parasympathetic nervous system** regulates the calmer functions (rest and digest) of our existence.

RECEPTORS AND NEUROTRANSMITTERS

Nerve endings of the sympathetic nervous system and the parasympathetic nervous system secrete neurotransmitters. The sympathetic nervous system has two types of **receptor** fibers at the nerve endings. The receptors are the alpha and beta receptors. The chemical neurotransmitter for the sympathetic nervous system is **norepinephrine**. These nerve endings are called **adrenergic**. When norepinephrine is released, an increase in heart rate and contractile force of cardiac fibers and vasoconstriction will result.

The chemical neurotransmitter for the parasympathetic nervous system is **acetylcholine**, and the nerve endings are known as **cholinergic**. When acetylcholine is released, the heart rate slows, as does the atrioventricular conduction rate. With the exception of capillaries, all the body's blood vessels have alpha-adrenergic receptors, whereas the heart and lungs have beta-adrenergic receptors.

sympathetic nervous system responsible for preparation of the body for physical activity (fight or flight)

parasympathetic nervous system regulates the calmer (rest and digest) functions

norepinephrine the chemical neurotransmitter for the sympathetic nervous system

acetylcholine the chemical neurotransmitter for the parasympathetic nervous system

Understanding adrenergic receptors and their effects on heart rate

For the sake of simplicity, we will discuss only the basics of the receptors and neurotransmitters. Let's first consider some rudimentary definitions:

Adrenergic—of or pertaining to the sympathetic nerve fibers of the autonomic nervous system that use epinephrine or epinephrine-like (norepinephrine) substances as neurotransmitters.

Receptor—reactive site on the cell surface or within the cell that combines with a drug molecule to produce a physiological effect.

Cholinergic—of or pertaining to the parasympathetic nerve fibers of the autonomic nervous system that use acetylcholine as the neurotransmitter.

The effects of the alpha- and beta-receptors are briefly described as follows (see also ■ **Table 2–1** and **Table 2–2**):

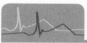

TABLE 2–1

Alpha		*Beta*	
Vasoconstriction	**Beta₁**	**Beta₂**	
Increase BP	Increase HR	Bronchial dilation	
	Increase contractility	Vasodilation	

Remember A B C D!

A B C D = *Alpha Constricts, Beta Dilates*

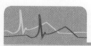

TABLE 2–2 Organs Affected by Alpha- and Beta-Receptors

Organs Affected	Alpha	Beta₁	Beta₂
Heart	Yes	Yes	No
Lungs	No	No	Yes
Vessels	Yes	No	Yes

CHAPTER 2

SUMMARY

It is important to understand not only the structure of the cardiovascular system, but also the function of the various structures. Indeed, it would be difficult to understand just why a particular component of the heart had ceased to function properly unless you were familiar with the proper, or "normal," function of that component. Thus, this chapter has focused on simplifying a very complicated subject—cardiovascular physiology.

KEY POINTS TO REMEMBER

1. The right atrium functions in part to receive unoxygenated blood from the head, neck, and trunk.
2. The right ventricle receives blood from the right atrium and pumps it to the pulmonary system.
3. The left atrium receives oxygenated blood from the pulmonary system.
4. The left ventricle receives this oxygenated blood from the left atrium and pumps it to the body system.
5. The cardiac cycle represents the time from initiation of ventricular contraction to initiation of the next ventricular contraction.
6. Systole (ventricular systole) is consistent with simultaneous contraction of the ventricles; diastole is synonymous with ventricular relaxation.
7. Stroke volume refers to the volume of blood pumped out of one ventricle of the heart in a single beat or contraction and is estimated at 70 cc per beat (or contraction).
8. Cardiac output is the amount of blood pumped by the left ventricle in 1 minute.

9. Also called end-diastolic pressure, preload is the pressure in the ventricles at the end of diastole; afterload is the resistance against which the heart must pump.
10. When the volume of blood in the ventricles is increased, stretching the ventricular myocardial fibers and consequently causing a more forceful contraction, a concept known as Starling's Law of the heart is the result.
11. The autonomic nervous system regulates functions of the body that are involuntary or are not under conscious control. Heart rate and blood pressure are regulated by this component of the nervous system.
12. There are two major divisions of the autonomic nervous system: the sympathetic nervous system and the parasympathetic nervous system.
13. The sympathetic nervous system is responsible for preparation of the body for physical activity (fight or flight).
14. The parasympathetic nervous system regulates the calmer (rest and digest) functions of our existence.

 ## REVIEW QUESTIONS

1. The left side of the heart is a low-pressure pump.
   a. True
   b. False

2. The major blood vessel that receives blood from the head and upper extremities and transports it to the heart is the:
   a. Trunk of the aorta
   b. Superior vena cava
   c. Inferior vena cava
   d. Pulmonary artery

3. The course of blood flow through the heart and lungs is referred to as _____ circulation.
   a. Aortic
   b. Pulmonary
   c. Systemic
   d. Collateral

4. Cardiac output is a factor of which of the following elements?
   a. Cardiac rate
   b. Stroke volume
   c. Partial vascular resistance
   d. Both a and b

5. The chief chemical neurotransmitter for the parasympathetic nervous system is:
   a. Acetylcholine
   b. Norepinephrine
   c. Epinephrine
   d. Atropine

6. It is important to note that blood vessels are innervated only by the _____ nervous system.
   a. Adrenergic
   b. Parasympathetic
   c. Sympathetic
   d. Cholinergic

7. The chief chemical neurotransmitter for the sympathetic nervous system is:
   a. Acetylcholine
   b. Norepinephrine
   c. Ephedrine
   d. Atropine

8. Unoxygenated blood flows from the inferior and superior vena cavae into the:
   a. Left atrium
   b. Left ventricle
   c. Right ventricle
   d. Right atrium

9. One cardiac cycle occurs every _____ seconds.
   a. 0.8 seconds   **c.** 0.52 seconds
   b. 0.5 seconds   **d.** 1.2 seconds

10. With the exception of _____, all the body's blood vessels have alpha-adrenergic receptors whereas the heart and lungs have beta-adrenergic receptors.
    a. Arterioles   **c.** Venules
    b. Capillaries   **d.** Aorta

11. Blood travels from the left atrium through the _____ valve and into the left ventricle.
    a. Aortic   **c.** Bicuspid
    b. Pulmonic   **d.** Tricuspid

12. Blood travels from the right atrium through the _____ valve and into the right ventricle.
    a. Aortic   **c.** Mitral
    b. Pulmonic   **d.** Tricuspid

13. Starling's Law of the heart is also referred to as:
    a. Cushing's theory
    b. Beck's triad
    c. The rubber band theory
    d. The Hering-Breuer reflex

14. Stroke volume is estimated at approximately _____ ml per beat.
    a. 40   **c.** 60
    b. 50   **d.** 70

15. The _____ nervous system is responsible for preparation of the body for physical activity (fight or flight).
    a. Sympathetic   **c.** Peripheral
    b. Parasympathetic   **d.** Adrenergic

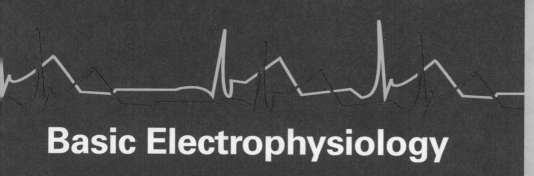

Basic Electrophysiology

INTRODUCTION

Although an in-depth study of cardiac electrophysiology can be quite complicated and baffling to the novice student, the intent of this text is to concentrate on the *basics* of interpreting dysrhythmias. Thus this discussion of electrophysiology will center on rudimentary, but very important, concepts.

In our discussion of cardiac anatomy in Chapter 1, we established that the heart is a unique and distinctive organ, unlike any other organ in the human body. The heart is composed of cardiac muscle, which is made up of thousands of myocardial cells. For the purposes of our discussion, we will note that there are two basic myocardial cell groups: the myocardial working cells and the specialized pacemaker cells of the electrical conduction system.

BASIC CELL GROUPS

Myocardial working cells

The **myocardial working cells** are responsible for generating the physical contraction of the heart muscle. The thin muscular layer of the wall of the atria and the thicker muscular layer of the ventricular walls are composed of myocardial working cells. Myocardial working cells are permeated by contractile filaments, which, when electrically stimulated, produce myocardial contraction. Thus the primary functions of the myocardial working cells include both contraction and relaxation.

It should be noted that this physical contraction of myocardial tissue actually generates blood flow; however, organized electrical activity is required in order to produce the physical contraction. As the myocardial tissue contracts, the size of the atria and ventricles decreases, so that blood is ejected from the chambers.

myocardial working cells responsible for generating the physical contraction of the heart muscle

Specialized pacemaker cells

Unlike the myocardial working cells, the specialized pacemaker cells of the electrical conduction system do not contain contractile filaments and thus do not have the ability to contract. Rather, the cells in this **specialized group** are responsible for controlling the rate and rhythm of the heart by coordinating regular depolarization. These cells are found in the electrical conduction system of the heart. Thus the generation and the conduction of electrical impulses are the primary functions of the specialized myocardial pacemaker cells. These cells have the ability to create an electrical impulse without being stimulated by a nerve.

Cardiac muscle cells have the ability to contract in response to thermal, chemical, electrical, or mechanical stimuli. All atrial muscle cells contract simultaneously; comparably, all ventricular muscle cells contract together.

specialized group responsible for controlling the rate and rhythm of the heart by coordinating regular depolarization and are found in the electrical conduction system of the heart

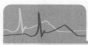

TABLE 3–1 Primary Cardiac Cell Characteristics

Characteristic	Location	Function
Automaticity	SA node, AV junction, Purkinje network fibers	Electrical
Excitability	All cardiac cells	Electrical
Conductivity	All cardiac cells	Electrical
Contractility	Myocardial muscle cells	Mechanical

threshold refers to the point at which a stimulus will produce a cell response

automaticity the ability of cardiac pacemaker cells to generate their own electrical impulses spontaneously without external (or nervous) stimulation

excitability the ability of cardiac cells to respond to an electrical stimulus, a characteristic shared by all cardiac cells

conductivity the ability of cardiac cells to receive an electrical stimulus and then transmit it to other cardiac cells

contractility (also referred to as rhythmicity) is the ability of cardiac cells to shorten and cause cardiac muscle contraction in response to an electrical stimulus

electrolyte a substance or compound whose molecules dissociate into charged components, or ions, when placed in water, producing positively and negatively charged ions

cation an ion with a positive charge

anion an ion with a negative charge

The term **threshold** refers to the point at which a stimulus will produce a cell response. When a stimulus is strong enough for cardiac cells to reach the threshold, all cells will respond to this stimulus and will thus contract. This action is known as the *all-or-none* phenomenon of cardiac muscle cells; that is, all cells will respond or none will respond. Hence, cardiac muscle functions on an all-or-none principle.

PRIMARY CARDIAC CELL CHARACTERISTICS

Cardiac cells have four primary cell characteristics. (See ■ **Table 3–1**.) These properties are excitability (or irritability), conductivity, contractility (or rhythmicity), and automaticity. Only one of these characteristics, contractility, is considered a mechanical function of the heart. The other three characteristics—automaticity, excitability, and conductivity—are electrical functions of the heart.

Automaticity is the ability of cardiac pacemaker cells to generate their own electrical impulses spontaneously without external (or nervous) stimulation. This intrinsic spontaneous depolarization frequency produces contraction of myocardial muscle cells. This characteristic is specific to the pacemaker cell sites of the electrical conduction system (i.e., the sinoatrial [SA] node, the atrioventricular [AV] junction, and the Purkinje network fibers which are discussed in Chapter 4).

Excitability—or irritability—is the ability of cardiac cells to respond to an electrical stimulus. This characteristic is shared by all cardiac cells. A weaker stimulus can cause a contraction when a cardiac cell is highly irritable.

Conductivity is the ability of cardiac cells to receive an electrical stimulus and then transmit it to other cardiac cells. This characteristic is shared by all cardiac cells because these cells are connected together to form a syncytium; that is, they function collectively as a unit. In referring to more than one of these units, the correct term is *syncytia*.

Contractility, also referred to as rhythmicity, is the ability of cardiac cells to shorten and cause cardiac muscle contraction in response to an electrical stimulus. Contractility can be thought of as the coordination of contractions of cardiac muscle cells to produce a regular heartbeat. Through the administration of certain medications, such as dopamine, digoxin, and epinephrine, cardiac contractility can be strengthened.

MAJOR ELECTROLYTES THAT AFFECT CARDIAC FUNCTION

Because myocardial cells are bathed in electrolyte solutions, both mechanical and electrical cardiac functions are influenced by electrolyte imbalances. An **electrolyte** is a substance or compound whose molecules dissociate into charged components, or *ions*, when placed in water, producing positively and negatively charged ions. An ion with a positive charge is called a **cation**, and an ion with a negative charge is called an **anion**.

The three major cations that affect cardiac function are potassium (K), sodium (Na), and calcium (Ca). Magnesium (Mg) is also an important cation. Phosphorus (P) and Chloride (Cl) are anions. Primarily, potassium (K), magnesium (Mg), and calcium (Ca) are intracellular (inside the cell) cations, whereas sodium is an extracellular (outside the cell) cation.

✳ Potassium performs a major function in cardiac depolarization and repolarization. An increase in potassium blood levels is known as hyperkalemia; a potassium deficit is hypokalemia.

✳ Sodium plays a vital part in depolarization of the myocardium. An increase in sodium blood levels is known as hypernatremia; a sodium deficit is hyponatremia.

✳ Calcium has an important function in myocardial depolarization and myocardial contraction. An increase in calcium blood levels is known as hypercalcemia; a calcium deficit is defined as hypocalcemia.

MOVEMENT OF IONS

Let's think now about the cardiac cells at rest, or in their resting state. Normally there is an ionic difference on the two sides of the cell membrane. In this state, potassium ion concentration is greater inside the cell than outside, and sodium ion concentration is greater outside the cell than inside. Potassium ions can diffuse through the membrane more readily than can sodium ions. By means of an active, or energized, mechanism of transport called the sodium-potassium exchange pump, potassium and sodium ions are moved in and out of the cell through the cell membrane. During the polarized, or resting, state, the inside of the cell is electrically negative relative to the outside of the cell. For the purposes of our discussions in the upcoming chapters, it should be noted that during this resting period a baseline or isoelectric line is recorded on the EKG (electrocardiogram) strip.

CARDIAC DEPOLARIZATION

When an impulse develops and spreads throughout the myocardium, certain changes occur in the heart muscle fibers. These changes are referred to as cardiac depolarization and cardiac repolarization. In order to interpret an EKG accurately and reasonably, one must understand the concept of cardiac depolarization and repolarization.

First, some terms (with definitions) that will be used in this discussion are as follows:

Resting membrane potential—state of a cardiac cell in which the inside of the cell membrane is negative compared with the outside of the cell membrane; exists when cardiac cells are in the resting state.

Action potential—change in polarity; a five-phase cycle that produces changes in the cell membrane's electrical charge; caused by stimulation of myocardial cells which extends across the myocardium; propagated in an all-or-none fashion.

Syncytium—cardiac muscle cell groups that are connected together and function collectively as a unit.

Polarized state—resting state of a cardiac cell, wherein the inside of the cell is electrically negative relative to the outside of the cell.

Permeability—the ability of the cell membrane to change to allow the movement of ions.

Depolarization—electrical occurrence normally expected to result in myocardial contraction; involves the movement of ions across cardiac cell membranes, resulting in positive polarity inside the cell membrane.

Repolarization—process whereby the depolarized cell is polarized and positive charges are again on the outside and negative charges on the inside of the cell; a return to the resting state.

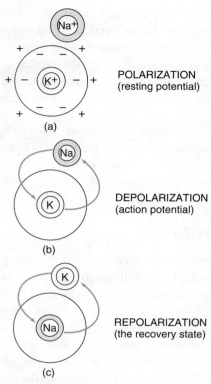

FIGURE 3–1. Ion shifts during depolarization and repolarization

For clarity, cardiac depolarization may be thought of as the period during which sodium ions rush into the cell, changing the interior charge to positive, after a myocardial cell has been stimulated. Recall now that this change of polarity is referred to as the action potential. In an effort to change the interior cell polarity to positive, calcium also slowly enters the cell. This activated state of the myocardial cells now spreads through the syncytium, followed closely by myocardial muscle contraction. This difference in the electric charge, or polarity, on the outside of the cell membrane results in the flow of electric current, which is recorded as waveforms on the EKG. (See ■ **Figure 3–1**.)

CARDIAC REPOLARIZATION

At the end of cardiac depolarization, the sodium actively returns to the outside of the cell, and potassium returns to the inside of the cell. This exchange takes place via the sodium-potassium exchange pump. The cell has now returned to the recovered, or repolarized, state. The cardiac cell is now ready to be stimulated again. Repolarization is a slower process than depolarization.

It may be helpful to recall that the polarized cell is in the resting state, the depolarized cell is utilizing its action potential, and the repolarized cell is in the recovery phase. It should be noted that the last area to be depolarized is the first area to be repolarized in normal, healthy cardiac muscle.

REFRACTORY PERIODS

Like all other excitable tissues, cardiac muscle tissue has a refractory period that attempts to ensure that the muscle is totally relaxed before another action potential or depolarization can be initiated. The refractory period of atrial muscle (approximately 0.15 sec) is much shorter than that of the ventricular muscle (approximately 0.25 to 0.3 sec). Thus the rate of atrial contractions can potentially be much faster than that of the ventricles.

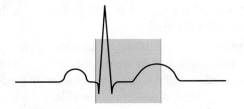

Absolute Refractory Period   Relative Refractory Period

FIGURE 3–2. Refractory periods

After electrical impulse stimulation and myocardial contraction, the cardiac cells have a brief resting period. As we learned earlier in this discussion, this period of rest is referred to as cardiac repolarization. During this state of repolarization, the heart goes through two stages: the absolute refractory period and the relative refractory period. (See ■ **Figure 3–2.**)

During most of the process of repolarization, the cardiac cell is unable to respond to a new electrical stimulus. In addition, the cardiac cell cannot spontaneously depolarize. This stage of cell activity is referred to as the **absolute refractory period**. Remember that, regardless of the strength of the stimulus, the cardiac cell cannot be stimulated to depolarize in this period. The absolute refractory period corresponds with the beginning of the QRS complex to the peak of the T wave on the EKG strip.

The second part of the refractory period follows the absolute refractory period and is referred to as the **relative refractory period**. This is the period when repolarization is almost complete, and the cardiac cell can be stimulated to contract prematurely if the stimulus is much stronger than normal. On the EKG strip, the relative refractory period corresponds with the downslope of the T wave. The relative refractory period is also known as the vulnerable period of the cardiac cells during repolarization.

absolute refractory period stage of cell activity in which the cardiac cell cannot spontaneously depolarize

relative refractory period the period when repolarization is almost complete, and the cardiac cell can be stimulated to contract prematurely if the stimulus is much stronger than normal

CHAPTER 3

SUMMARY

As you began to comprehend through your study of Chapters 1 and 2, the heart is a unique organ, unlike any other organ in the human body. You should now understand that the heart is composed of cardiac muscle made up of thousands of myocardial cells. In this chapter, we discussed the two basic myocardial cell groups: the myocardial working cells and the specialized pacemaker cells of the electrical conduction system.

KEY POINTS TO REMEMBER

1. The myocardial working cells are responsible for generating the physical contraction of the heart muscle.

2. The specialized pacemaker cells are responsible for controlling the rate and rhythm of the heart by coordinating regular depolarization. These cells are found in the electrical conduction system of the heart.

3. Automaticity is the ability of cardiac pacemaker cells to spontaneously generate their own electrical impulses without external (or nervous) stimulation.

4. Excitability is the ability of cardiac cells to respond to an electrical stimulus. This characteristic is shared by all cardiac cells and is referred to as irritability.

5. Conductivity is the ability of cardiac cells to receive an electrical stimulus and to then transmit the stimulus to other cardiac cells.

6. Contractility is referred to as rhythmicity and is the ability of cardiac cells to shorten and cause cardiac muscle contraction in response to an electrical stimulus.

7. Potassium performs a major function in cardiac depolarization and repolarization.

8. Sodium plays a vital part in depolarization of the myocardium.

9. Calcium renders an important function in myocardial depolarization and contraction.

10. When the cardiac cell is at rest, the potassium ion concentration is greater inside the cell than outside and sodium ion concentration is greater outside the cell than inside.

11. By means of an active mechanism of transport called the sodium-potassium exchange pump, potassium and sodium ions are moved in and out of the cell through the cell membrane.

12. Depolarization is an electrical occurrence resulting in myocardial contraction involving the movement of ions across cardiac cell membranes, resulting in positive polarity inside the cell membrane. Repolarization is a process whereby the depolarized cell is polarized, and positive charges are again on the outside and negative charges are on the inside of the cell. Repolarization is a return to the resting state.

13. During the majority of the process of repolarization, the cardiac cell is unable to respond to a new electrical stimulus; the cardiac cell cannot spontaneously depolarize, and this period is referred to as the absolute refractory period.

14. The relative refractory period is the period when repolarization is almost complete and the cardiac cell can be stimulated to contract prematurely if the stimulus is much stronger than normal.

15. On the EKG strip, the relative refractory period corresponds with the downslope of the T wave and is called the vulnerable period of repolarization.

REVIEW QUESTIONS

1. The primary functions of the myocardial working cells include:
   a. Automaticity
   b. Regeneration
   c. Contraction and relaxation
   d. Impulse propagation

2. The ability of cardiac pacemaker cells to generate their own electrical impulses spontaneously without external, or nervous, stimulation is known as:
   a. Automaticity c. Conductility
   b. Contractility d. Action potential

3. Which characteristic is specific to the pacemaker sites of the electrical conduction system (i.e., the SA node, the AV junction, and the Purkinje network fibers)?
   a. Automaticity c. Conductility
   b. Contractility d. Excitability

4. The ability of cardiac cells to respond to an electrical stimulus is referred to as:
   a. Automaticity c. Conductility
   b. Contractility d. Excitability

5. Excitability is also referred to as:
   a. Irritability c. Contractility
   b. Automaticity d. Conductility

6. The ability of cardiac cells to receive an electrical stimulus and then transmit the stimulus to other cardiac cells is known as:
   a. Irritability c. Contractility
   b. Automaticity d. Conductivity

7. Conductivity is a characteristic shared by all cardiac cells.
   a. True b. False

8. Cardiac muscle cell groups that function collectively as a unit are known as:
   a. Syncytia   c. Electrical
   b. Refractory   d. Bundles

9. Repolarization is a slower process than depolarization.
   a. True   b. False

10. The period when repolarization is almost complete and the cardiac cell can be stimulated to contract prematurely if the stimulus is stronger than normal is known as:
    a. The relative refractory period
    b. The absolute refractory period
    c. The action potential phase
    d. Absolute depolarization

11. Cardiac depolarization may be thought of as the period during which _____ ions rush into the cell.
    a. Potassium   c. Sodium
    b. Calcium   d. Chloride

myocardium depolarization

12. At the end of cardiac depolarization, _____ ions return to the inside of the cell.
    a. Potassium   c. Sodium
    b. Calcium   d. Magnesium

13. The resting state of a cardiac cell, wherein the inside of the cell is electrically negative relative to the outside of the cell, is called:
    a. Active state   c. Depolarization
    b. Polarized state   d. Repolarization

14. The point at which a stimulus will produce a cell response is called the:
    a. Active state   c. Threshold
    b. All-or-none phase d. Rest state

15. An increase in potassium blood levels is known as:
    a. Hypernatremia   c. Hypercalcemia
    b. Hypokalemia   d. Hyperkalemia

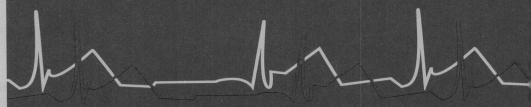

4

Objectives

Upon completion of this chapter, the student will be able to:

- Identify the location of the following:

  a. Sinoatrial node

  b. Internodal pathways

  c. Bachmann's bundle

  d. Atrioventricular node

  e. Bundle of His

  f. Atrioventricular junction

  g. Bundle branches

  h. Purkinje's network

- Discuss the function of the each of the components listed below:

  a. SA node

  b. Internodal pathways

  c. Bachmann's bundle

  d. AV node

  e. Bundle of His

  f. AV Junction

  g. Bundle branches

  h. Purkinje's network

- Explain the normal path of an impulse traveling through the electrical conduction system

The Electrical Conduction System

INTRODUCTION

The heart's pacing, or conduction, system is responsible for the electrical activity that controls each normal heartbeat. This unique system consists of specialized cells and fibers that are collectively known as nodes or bundles. These nodes and bundles are relatively small and are located primarily beneath the endocardium (the innermost lining of the chambers of the heart). Specialized parts of this system are capable of initiating electrical activity automatically and can act as pacemakers for the heart. (See ■ **Figure 4–1** and ■ **Table 4–1**.)

A thorough understanding of the electrical conduction system of the heart is an essential component of learning and understanding an electrocardiogram (EKG) strip. While it is important to note that the EKG strip itself is representative of only the electrical activity of the heart, the student must also understand that the clinician cannot determine the mechanical activity of a patient's heart by merely looking at an EKG strip.

In order to begin to determine that an EKG strip is "abnormal," the student must first understand the normal parameters for the graphic representation of the electrical activity of the heart. It is to that end that this chapter is presented. In this chapter, you will learn where the pacemakers and conducting fibers are located, as well as how they function during a normal heartbeat.

SINOATRIAL NODE

The sinoatrial (SA) node is located in the upper posterior portion of the right atrial wall of the heart, near the opening of the superior vena cava. The node is made up of a cluster of hundreds of different types of cells that comprise a knot of modified heart muscle. It is generally believed that slightly fewer than 50 percent of the cells are actual pacemaker cells, whereas the majority of the remaining cells function to conduct the electrical impulse within the SA node. This cluster is capable of generating impulses that travel throughout the muscle fibers of both atria, resulting in depolarization.

As discussed in Chapter 2, heart rate and blood pressure are regulated by the autonomic nervous system. An increase in the rate of firing of the SA node—that is, increased heart rate—may occur as a result of stimulation of the sympathetic nervous system. A clear example of a causative factor that provokes an increase in heart rate is exercise; conversely, if the vagus nerve is stimulated, the heart rate will decrease. The parasympathetic nervous system regulates the calmer functions of our existence.

The SA node primarily receives its blood supply from the SA artery. The SA artery is a branch of the right coronary artery in approximately 60 percent to 70 percent of the population. However, in approximately 30 percent to 40 percent of the population, the circumflex artery supplies blood to the SA node.

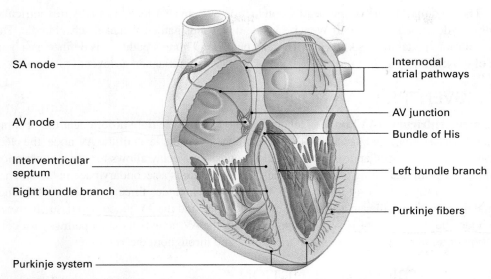

SA node

AV node

Interventricular
septum

Right bundle branch

Purkinje system

Internodal
atrial pathways

AV junction

Bundle of His

Left bundle branch

Purkinje fibers

FIGURE 4–1. Cardiac conduction system

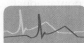

TABLE 4–1 Review of the Electrical Conduction System of the Heart

SA Node	Internodal Pathways	AV Junction, AV Node, and Bundle	Bundle Branches	Purkinje's Network
Firing rate 60–100 BPM	Transfer impulse from the SA node throughout the atria to the AV junction	Slows impulse intrinsic firing rate of 40–60 BPM	Two main branches (left and right) transmit impulse to ventricles	Spreads impulse throughout the ventricles; intrinsic firing rate 20–40 BPM

The **SA node** is commonly referred to as the primary pacemaker of the heart because it normally depolarizes more rapidly than any other part of the conduction system. The normal range, or firing rate, of the heart's primary pacemaker (the SA node) is 60 to 100 beats per minute (BPM).

If, for any of a variety of reasons, the dominant pacemaker fails to fire within the normal range, another group of specialized tissues, such as the atrioventricular (AV) tissue or the Purkinje network of fibers, will assume the duties of the pacemaker. These backup pacemakers are arranged in a waterfall fashion. Depolarization and resultant myocardial contraction occur as the impulse leaves the SA node and travels further down the path of the electrical conduction system.

INTERNODAL PATHWAYS

Three **internodal tracts**, or pathways, receive the electrical impulse as it leaves the SA node. These tracts distribute the electrical impulse throughout the atrial muscle and transmit the impulse from the SA node to the AV node. The internodal tracts consist of anterior, middle, and posterior divisions, or Bachmann's bundle, Wenckebach's bundle, and Thorel's pathway.

BACHMANN'S BUNDLE, WENCKEBACH'S BUNDLE, AND THOREL'S PATHWAY

Bachmann's bundle is a group of interatrial fibers contained in the left atrium. It is a subdivision of the anterior internodal tract, respectively. There are, in reality, two branches of the anterior internodal tract, Bachmann's bundle plus a descending branch. This specialized group of cardiac fibers conducts electrical activity from the SA node to the left atrium.

SA node commonly referred to as the primary pacemaker of the heart because it normally depolarizes more rapidly than any other part of the conduction system

internodal tracts distribute the electrical impulse throughout the atria and transmit the impulse from the SA node to the AV node

Bachmann's bundle a subdivision of the anterior internodal tract, conducts electrical activity from the SA node to the left atrium

The medium bundle of the heart's conduction system that leads to the Atrioventricular node was described by Dr. Karl Wenckebach and was thus named Wenckebach's bundle. The posterior internodal tract is known as Thorel's pathway. Thorel's pathway is defined as a bundle of muscle fibers in the human heart connecting the sinoatrial and atrioventricular nodes.

ATRIOVENTRICULAR NODE

atrioventricular (AV) node located on the floor of the right atrium near the opening of the coronary sinus and just above the tricuspid valve; at the level of the AV node, the electrical activity is delayed approximately 0.05 seconds

AV junction the region where the AV node joins the bundle of His

The **atrioventricular (AV) node** is located on the floor of the right atrium near the opening of the coronary sinus and just above the tricuspid valve. At the level of the AV node, the electrical activity is delayed approximately 0.05 seconds. This delay allows for atrial contraction and a more complete filling of the ventricles. The AV node is a secondary pacemaker and has an intrinsic firing rate of 40 to 60 BPM. The AV node includes three regions: the AV junctional tissue between the atria and node, the nodal area, and the AV junctional tissue between the node and the bundle of His. In the typical heart, the AV node is the only pathway for conduction of atrial electrical impulses to travel into and throughout the ventricles.

ATRIOVENTRICULAR JUNCTION

The region where the AV node joins the bundle of His is called the **AV junction**. Similar to the SA node, the AV junctional tissue contains fibers that can depolarize spontaneously, forming an electrical impulse that can spread to the heart chambers. Therefore, if the SA node fails or slows below its normal range, the AV junctional tissues can initiate electrical activity and thus assume the role of a secondary pacemaker. A concept called dominance is where the fastest pacemaker assumes control of the rate of depolarization of the atrium and ventricles. The electrical impulse is slowed in the AV node to allow the atria to empty in the ventricles before the ventricles contract.

If, on occasion, an impulse fails to follow the normal route, an accessory pathway may occur. An accessory pathway, sometimes called a bypass tract, may be defined as an irregular muscle connection between the atria and the ventricles that bypasses the AV node.

BUNDLE OF HIS

bundle of His the conduction pathway that leads out of the AV node and is also traditionally referred to as the common bundle

The conduction pathway that leads out of the AV node was described by a German physician, Wilhelm His, in 1893 and has subsequently been referred to as the **bundle of His**. This bundle receives its blood supply from the left anterior and posterior descending coronary arteries. The bundle of His is also referred to as the atrioventricular bundle or the common bundle. It is approximately 15 millimeters (mm) long and lies at the top of the interventricular septum, the wall between the right and left ventricles.

This bundle of specialized cells contains pacemaker cells that have the ability to self-initiate electrical activity. It also serves as the connection between the upper and lower chambers of the heart—the atria and ventricles.

BUNDLE BRANCHES

bundle branches two main branches, the right bundle branch and the left bundle branch, conduct electrical activity from the bundle of His down to the Purkinje network

The bundle of His divides into two main branches at the top of the interventricular septum. These branches are the right bundle branch and the left bundle branch. The primary function of the **bundle branches** is to conduct electrical activity from the bundle of His down to the Purkinje network. A long, thin structure lying beneath the endocardium, the right bundle branch runs down the right side of the interventricular septum and terminates at the papillary muscles in the right ventricle. This bundle branch functions to carry electrical impulses to the right ventricle.

Shorter than the right bundle branch, the left bundle branch divides into pathways that spread from the left side of the interventricular septum and throughout the left ventricle. The two main divisions of the left bundle branch are called fascicles. The anterior fascicle carries electrical impulses to the anterior wall of the left ventricle, and the posterior fascicle spreads the impulses to the posterior ventricular wall. The bundle branches continue to divide until they finally terminate in the Purkinje fibers.

PURKINJE'S NETWORK

Bundle branches lead to a network of small conduction fibers that spread throughout the ventricles. These fibers were first described in 1787 by Johannes E. Purkinje, a Czechoslovakian physiologist. This network of fibers carries electrical impulses directly to ventricular muscle cells. The fibers that connect with Purkinje's fibers start in the AV node in the right atrium of the heart. (See ■ **Figure 4–2.**)

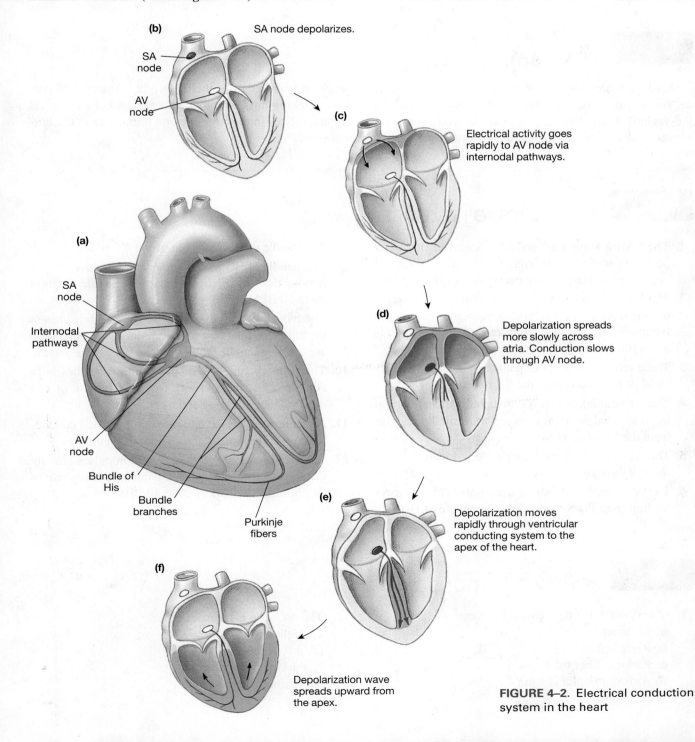

(b) SA node depolarizes.

SA node

AV node

(c) Electrical activity goes rapidly to AV node via internodal pathways.

(a)

SA node

Internodal pathways

AV node

Bundle of His

Bundle branches

Purkinje fibers

(d) Depolarization spreads more slowly across atria. Conduction slows through AV node.

(e) Depolarization moves rapidly through ventricular conducting system to the apex of the heart.

(f)

Depolarization wave spreads upward from the apex.

FIGURE 4–2. Electrical conduction system in the heart

Purkinje's network
a network of fibers that carries electrical impulses directly to ventricular muscle cells

Purkinje's network of fibers can only be identified with the aid of a microscope, but these fibers are larger in diameter than ordinary cardiac muscle fibers. Ventricular contraction is facilitated by the rapid spread of the electrical impulse through the left and right bundle branches and Purkinje fibers, into the ventricular muscle. Purkinje's network fibers possess the intrinsic ability to serve as a pacemaker. The firing rate of the Purkinje pacemaker fibers is normally within the range of 20 to 40 BPM.

CHAPTER 4

 ## SUMMARY

A thorough understanding of the heart's normal electrical conduction system is vital to your understanding of the various heart rhythms. In order to understand the causes of dysrhythmias, it is imperative that you have a working knowledge of the underlying concepts of normal sinus rhythm. As you now understand, the electrical impulse arises in the SA node and terminates in the Purkinje network.

 ## KEY POINTS TO REMEMBER

1. The SA (or sinoatrial) node is located in the upper posterior portion of the right atrial wall of the heart and serves as the primary pacemaker of the heart.

2. The SA node generates impulses that travel throughout the muscle fibers of both atria, resulting in depolarization; the intrinsic firing rate of the SA node is 60 to 100 BPM.

3. Three internodal tracts or pathways receive the electrical impulse as it exits the SA node.

4. The internodal pathways distribute the electrical impulse throughout the atria and transmit the impulse from the SA node to the AV node.

5. The AV (or atrioventricular) node is located on the floor of the right atrium just above the tricuspid valve.

6. The AV junction is where the internodal pathways leading from the SA node join the bundle of His.

7. The bundle of His leads out of the AV node.

8. The bundle of His may be referred to as the common bundle; the intrinsic firing rate of the bundle of His is 40 to 60 BPM.

9. The bundle of His divides into two main branches at the top of the interventricular septum. Those branches are the right bundle branch and the left bundle branch.

10. The primary function of the bundle branches is to conduct electrical activity from the bundle of His down to the Purkinje network.

11. Purkinje fibers make up a network of small conduction fibers that spread throughout the ventricles.

12. The Purkinje fibers carry electrical impulses directly to ventricular muscle cells; the intrinsic firing rate of the Purkinje network is 20 to 40 BPM.

 ## REVIEW QUESTIONS

1. The sinoatrial node is located in the:
   a. Right atrium
   b. Right ventricle
   c. Purkinje fiber tract
   d. Atrioventricular septum

2. The AV node is located in the:
   a. Right atrium
   b. Left ventricle
   c. Purkinje fiber tract
   d. Atrioventricular septum

3. The intrinsic firing rate of the AV junction is
   _____ BPM.
   a. 15–20   c. 35–45
   b. 25–35   d. 40–60

4. The intrinsic firing rate of the SA node is _____
   BPM.
   a. 20–60   c. 60–100
   b. 40–80   d. 80–100

5. The electrocardiogram is used to:
   a. Determine pulse rate
   b. Detect valvular dysfunction
   c. Evaluate electrical activity in the heart
   d. Determine whether the heart is beating

6. The normal conduction pattern of the heart follows
   the sequence:
   1. SA node
   2. Purkinje fibers
   3. Bundle of His
   4. AV node
   5. Bundle branches
   6. Internodal pathways
   a. 1, 2, 3, 5, 6, 4
   b. 1, 6, 4, 3, 5, 2
   c. 1, 6, 4, 2, 3, 5
   d. 6, 1, 5, 4, 3, 2

7. The intrinsic firing rate of the Purkinje network is
   _____ BPM.
   a. 60–80   c. 20–40
   b. 40–60   d. 10–20

8. The SA node receives its blood supply primarily
   from the:
   a. Left coronary artery
   b. Great cardiac vein
   c. Right coronary artery
   d. Aorta

9. _____ internodal tracts or pathways receive the
   electrical impulse as it leaves the SA node. These
   tracts distribute the electrical impulse throughout
   the atria and transmit the impulse from the SA node
   to the AV node.
   a. Two   c. Four
   b. Three   d. Five

10. What is the specialized group of cardiac fibers con-
    ducting electrical activity from the SA node to the
    left atrium?
    a. Purkinje network
    b. Bundle of His
    c. Bachmann's bundle
    d. Intercalated disks

11. The interventricular septum is the wall between the:
    a. Right and left atrium
    b. Right and left ventricle
    c. Inferior and superior chambers
    d. Inferior and superior vena cavae

12. Purkinje's network fibers can be identified only
    with the aid of a microscope.
    a. True   b. False

13. Purkinje's network fibers are smaller in diameter
    than ordinary cardiac muscle fibers.
    a. True   b. False

14. The primary functions of the myocardial working
    cells include:
    a. Automaticity
    b. Regeneration
    c. Contraction and relaxation
    d. Impulse propagation

15. The major blood vessel that receives blood from the
    systemic circulation is the:
    a. Superior vena cava   c. Inferior vena cava
    b. Great cardiac vein   d. Pulmonary artery

5

Objectives

Upon completion of this chapter, the student will be able to:

- Define the term electrocardiogram

- Discuss the basics of EKG monitoring

- List the types of EKG leads

- Discuss the relevance of Einthoven's triangle

- Identify and explain the grids and markings on a representative strip of EKG graph paper

- Describe the relationship of the following EKG waveforms to the electrical events in the heart:

    a. P wave

    b. PR interval

    c. QRS complex

    d. ST segment

    e. T wave

The Electrocardiogram

INTRODUCTION

The medical use of the electrocardiogram dates back to less than a century ago, around the year 1900. The equipment used at that time was large, cumbersome, and certainly not appropriate for use in small or confined spaces. Modern technology has brought us very far in the past 100 years, to the point where every emergency department and prehospital advanced life support unit has equipment suitable for obtaining an EKG on a patient whenever and wherever indicated. You will find that the most significant lesson to be learned as you travel throughout this textbook is to center not on the EKG tracing, but rather on the clinical picture of your patient. You must continually ask yourself: How is this rhythm clinically significant to the patient? Regardless of the pattern observed on the oscilloscope, your patient's condition is, and must be, your primary concern. Keep this important fact in mind, and your patient's best interest will always be served.

THE ELECTROCARDIOGRAM

electrocardiogram graphic representation of the electrical activity of the heart

The **electrocardiogram** (EKG or ECG—both abbreviations are acceptable) is a noninvasive procedure and is commonly defined as a graphic representation of the electrical activity of the heart. (See ■ **Figure 5–1**.) The term electrocardiogram originally came from the Greek terms "electro," related to electrical activity, "kardio," which relates to the word "heart," and "graph," which refers to the art of writing. The machine used to record the electrocardiogram is called an **electrocardiograph**, or, more simply, an EKG machine.

electrocardiograph machine used to record the electrocardiogram

Although EKG analysis serves as a useful diagnostic tool, the health care professional must be cognizant of the fact that the EKG is a graphic tracing of the *electrical activity* of the heart but not the *mechanical activity*. Thus, while much worthwhile information can be obtained from an EKG strip, there is certain valuable information that cannot be gleaned from the strip alone.

■ **Table 5–1** depicts the information that can and cannot be obtained from the analysis of an EKG strip.

ELECTRICAL BASIS OF THE EKG

In Chapter 4, we explored the components and functions of the heart's electrical conduction system. On the basis of that knowledge, we should understand that the heart generates electrical activity in the body; thus the body can be thought of as a major conductor of electrical activity. This electrical activity can be sensed by electrodes placed on the skin surface and can be recorded in the form of an electrocardiogram. Cardiac monitors depict the heart's electrical impulses as patterns

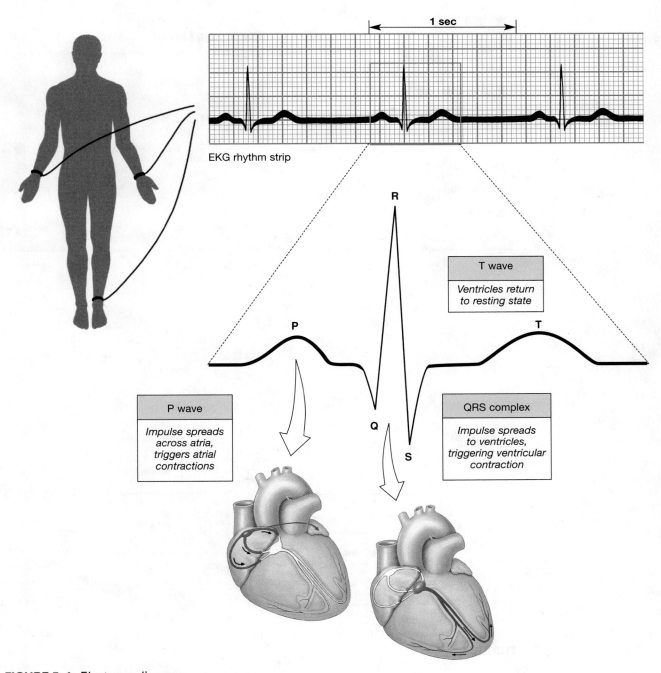

FIGURE 5–1. Electrocardiogram

of waves on the monitor screen or oscilloscope. Because electrical impulses present on the skin surface are of very low voltage, the impulses must be amplified by the EKG machine. The printed record of the electrical activity of the heart is called a **rhythm strip** or an **EKG strip**. (See ■ **Figure 5–2.**)

EKG LEADS

As we discussed earlier in this chapter, the cardiac monitor receives electrical impulses from the patient's heart through electrodes placed on particular areas of the body. An **electrode** is an adhesive pad that contains conductive gel and is designed to be attached to the patient's

rhythm strip or EKG strip the printed record of the electrical activity of the heart

electrode an adhesive pad that contains conductive gel and is designed to be attached to the patient's skin

TABLE 5–1 Information obtainable from EKG strip analysis

Heart rate	Yes	
Rhythm or regularity	Yes	
Impulse conduction time intervals	Yes	
Abnormal conduction pathways	Yes	
Pumping action		No
Cardiac output		No
Blood pressure		No
Cardiac muscle hypertrophy		No

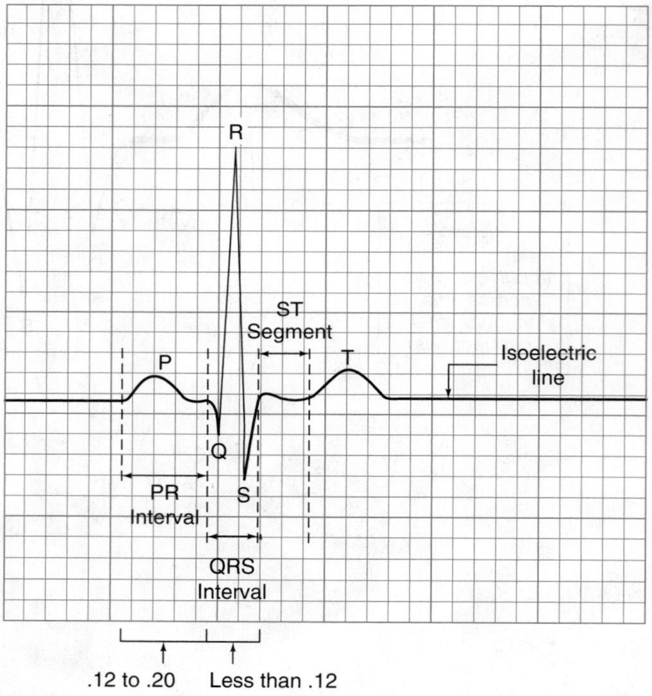

FIGURE 5–2. EKG

leads electrodes connected to the monitor or EKG machine by wires

Lead a pair of electrodes such as chest Lead I, II, MCL

skin. The electrodes are then connected to the monitor or EKG machine by wires called **leads**. These wires are generally color coded in order to be user-friendly.

In EKG monitoring, the term **Lead** is sometimes used in two different contexts. We use the other meaning of the term when speaking of a pair of electrodes: chest Lead I, II, MCL (modified chest lead), and so on. In this usage, the term is generally capitalized.

For the monitor or EKG machine to receive a clear picture of the electrical impulses generated by the heart's electrical conduction system, there must be a positive, a negative, and a ground lead. The ground lead serves to minimize outside electrical interference. The exact portion of the heart being visualized depends, in large part, on the placement of electrodes.

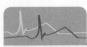

TABLE 5–2 Placement of bipolar leads

Lead	Positive Electrode	Negative Electrode
I	Left arm	Right arm
II	Left leg	Right arm
III	Left leg	Left arm

It may be helpful to envision the heart as an object placed on a pedestal, around which a person can move while taking photographs (different views) from all angles. This analogy would describe the 12-lead EKG, whereas only one snapshot or view of the heart would represent the 3-lead EKG. The 12-lead EKG is commonly used in hospitals and clinics; the 3-lead EKG is typically used in the field. It should be noted that some of the newer monitors require a fourth lead, which represents the right leg, while in most hospital settings, an additional fifth lead is utilized to monitor V_1, V_2, or V_3 chest leads. In some areas of the country, 12-lead EKGs are being used regularly to aid in screening patients who are potential candidates for percutaneous coronary intervention (PCI) or fibrinolytic (thrombolytic) therapy. It is important to note that the 3-lead EKG is sufficient for detecting life-threatening **dysrhythmias**, or abnormal heart rhythms.

Lead II and the MCL are most commonly used for cardiac monitoring because of their ability to visualize P waves. Chest Leads I, II, and III are known as **bipolar leads**, which means that these leads have one positive electrode and one negative electrode. Bipolar leads are sometimes referred to as limb leads. ■ **Table 5–2** represents the placement of electrodes of the three bipolar leads on certain areas of the body.

An imaginary inverted triangle is formed around the heart by proper placement of the bipolar leads. This triangle is referred to as Einthoven's triangle. (See ■ **Figure 5–3**.) The top of the triangle is formed by Lead I, the right side of the triangle is formed by Lead II, and the left side of the triangle is formed by Lead III. Each lead represents a different look at, or view, of the heart. For the sake of consistency, chest Lead II will be used throughout this textbook, except where otherwise designated.

dysrhythmias abnormal heart rhythms

bipolar leads have one positive electrode and one negative electrode

EKG GRAPH PAPER

Electrocardiographic paper (■ **Figure 5–4**) is arranged as a series of horizontal and vertical lines printed on graph paper and provides a printed record of cardiac electrical activity. This paper is standardized to allow for consistency in analyzing EKG rhythm strips. EKG paper leaves the machine at a constant speed of 25 millimeters per second (mm/sec).

Both time and amplitude (or voltage) are measured on graph paper. Time is measured on the horizontal line; amplitude or voltage is measured on the vertical line. The vertical axis reflects millivolts (mV); two large squares equal 1 mV. EKG graph paper is divided into small squares, each of which is 1 mm in height and width and represents a time interval of 0.04 seconds. Darker lines further divide the paper every fifth square, both vertically and horizontally. Each of these large squares measures 5 mm in height and 5 mm in width and represents a time interval of 0.20 seconds. There are five small squares in each large square. Therefore, 5 small squares × 0.04 seconds = 0.20 seconds. The squares on the EKG paper represent the measurement of the length of time required for the electrical impulse to traverse a specific part of the heart. Proper interpretation of EKG rhythms is dependent in part, on the understanding of the time increments as represented on EKG paper (Figure 5–4).

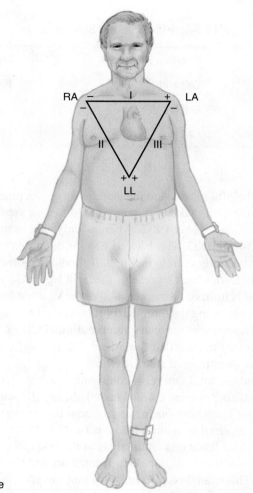

FIGURE 5–3. Einthoven's triangle

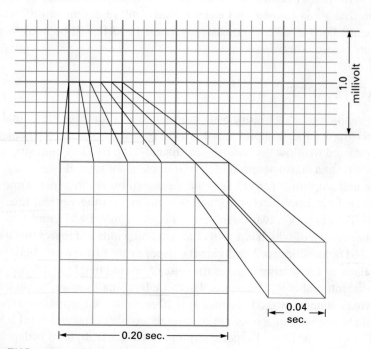

FIGURE 5–4. EKG paper and markings

EKG WAVEFORMS

A wave or waveform recorded on an EKG strip refers to movement away from the baseline, or isoelectric line, and is represented as a positive deflection (above the isoelectric line) or as a negative deflection (below the isoelectric line). The **baseline** is the straight line seen on an EKG strip; it represents the beginning and end point of all waves.

As the electrical impulse leaves the sinoatrial (SA) node, **EKG waveforms** are produced on the graph paper. One complete cardiac cycle is represented on graph paper by five major waves: the P wave; the Q, R, and S waves (normally referred to as the QRS complex); and the T wave.

P wave

As we discussed in Chapter 4, the SA node fires first during a normal cardiac cycle. This "firing" event sends the electrical impulse outward to stimulate both atria and manifests as the P wave. (See ■ **Figure 5–5**.) When observed on a Lead II EKG strip, the **P wave** is a smooth, rounded-upward deflection. The P wave represents depolarization of the left and right atria and is approximately 0.10 seconds in length.

PR interval

The **PR interval** (■ **Figure 5–6**), sometimes abbreviated PRI, represents the time interval necessary for the impulse to travel from the SA node through the internodal pathways in the atria and downward to the ventricles. In simpler terms, the PRI is said to represent the distance from the beginning of the P wave to the beginning of the QRS complex. The normal PR interval is measured as 3 to 5 small squares of the EKG graph paper and is 0.12 to 0.20 seconds in length.

baseline (isoelectric line): the straight line seen on an EKG strip; it represents the beginning and end point of all waves

EKG waveforms a wave or waveform recorded on an EKG strip refers to movement away from the baseline or isoelectric line and is represented as a positive deflection (above the isoelectric line) or as a negative deflection (below the isoelectric line)

P wave represents depolarization of the left and right atria

PR interval represents the time interval necessary for the impulse to travel from the SA node through the internodal pathways in the atria and downward to the ventricles

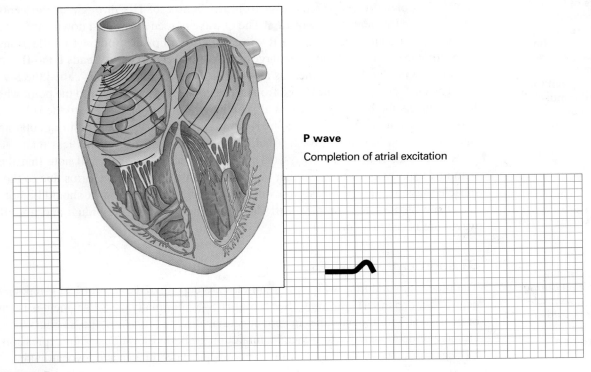

P wave

Completion of atrial excitation

FIGURE 5–5. P wave

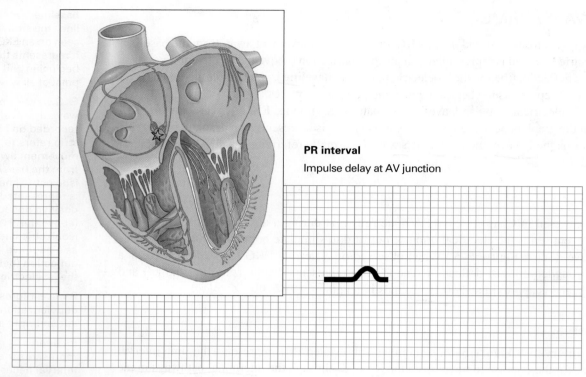

PR interval

Impulse delay at AV junction

FIGURE 5–6. PR interval

QRS complex

QRS complex
consists of the Q, R,
and S waves and
represents the
conduction of the
electrical impulse
from the bundle of
His throughout the
ventricular muscle,
or ventricular
depolarization

The **QRS complex** (■ **Figure 5–7**) consists of the Q, R, and S waves and represents the conduction of the electrical impulse from the bundle of His throughout the ventricular muscle, or ventricular depolarization. The Q wave is seen as the first downward (negative) deflection following the PRI. The R wave is the first upward (positive) deflection of the QRS complex and is normally the largest deflection seen in chest Leads I and II. Immediately following the R wave, there is a downward deflection, which is called the S wave.

The QRS complex is measured from the beginning of the Q wave to the point where the S wave meets the baseline. There is also an interval from one R wave to the subsequent R wave and this interval is known as the R-R interval, most often utilized in calculating heart rates (discussed in Chapter 6). Normally, the QRS complex measures less than 0.12 seconds or less than three small squares on EKG graph paper. You will note that the QRS complex usually has a much higher amplitude than the other waveforms due to the larger muscle mass of the ventricles versus the smaller mass of the atria. It should be noted that the shape of the QRS complex will vary from individual to individual and not all three waves are necessarily present.

ST segment

ST segment the
time interval during
which the ventricles
are depolarized and
ventricular
repolarization
begins

The time interval during which the ventricles are depolarized and ventricular repolarization begins is called the **ST segment**. (See ■ **Figure 5–8**.) Normally the ST segment is isoelectric, or consistent with the baseline. In certain cardiac disease processes, the ST segment may be elevated or depressed due to ischemia, infarction, or both. Elevation and/or depression of the ST segment is one of the major EKG changes appreciated in an acute myocardial infarction.

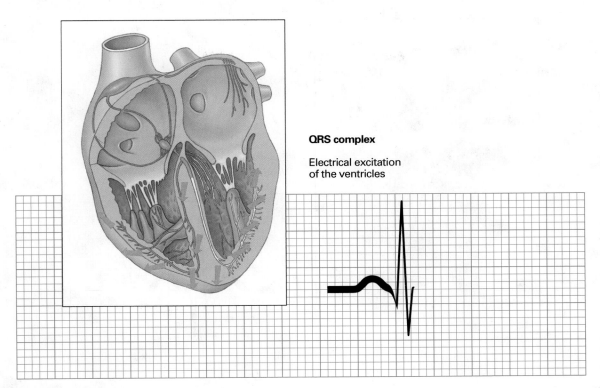

QRS complex

Electrical excitation
of the ventricles

FIGURE 5–7. QRS complex

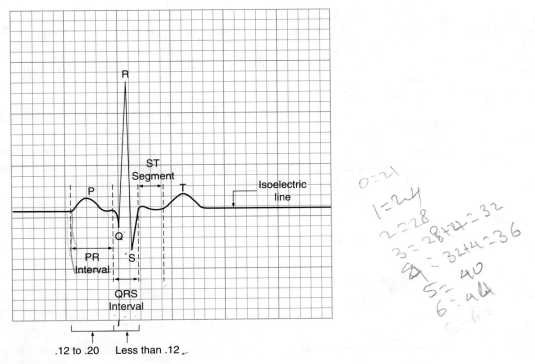

FIGURE 5–8. EKG waveforms

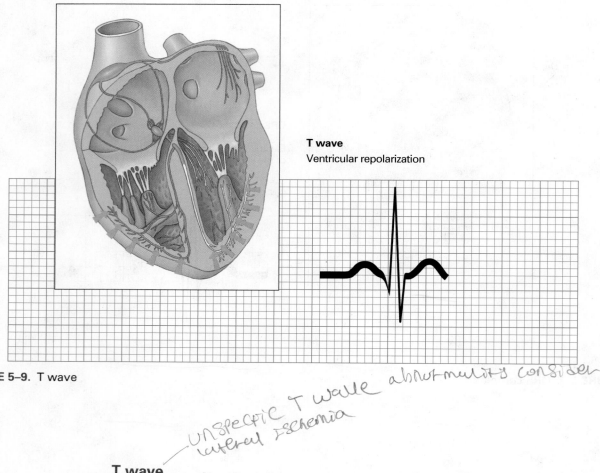

T wave
Ventricular repolarization

FIGURE 5–9. T wave

unspecific T wave abnormality consider lateral Ischemia

T wave

T wave represents ventricular repolarization and follows the ST segment

Following the ST segment is the **T wave** (**Figure 5–9**), which represents ventricular repolarization. The T wave is normally seen as a slightly asymmetrical, slightly rounded, positive deflection. Recall now that ventricular repolarization is an electrical event with no associated activity of the ventricular musculature. The T wave is often referred to as the *resting phase* of the cardiac cycle.

Recall also that the refractory periods, both absolute and relative, are in place during the EKG representation of the T wave; thus the heart may be vulnerable to strong impulses, which may lead to ventricular dysrhythmias. The T wave may be either elevated or depressed in the presence of current or previous cardiac ischemia. Normally, one complete cardiac cycle is represented by the P-QRS-T pattern. (See **Table 5–3**.)

TABLE 5–3 Summary of EKG waveforms and correlating cardiac events

P wave represents	Atrial depolarization
QRS complex represents	Ventricular depolarization; atrial repolarization
T wave represents	Ventricular repolarization

CHAPTER 5

 SUMMARY

Now that we have discussed the components of the electrocardiogram, let me remind you that it is imperative always, at all times, to **observe and treat the patient on the basis of his or her clinical presentation, regardless** **of the rhythm being observed on the oscilloscope!** Always remember to ask yourself: How is this rhythm clinically significant to my patient? (See ■ **Figure 5–10.**)

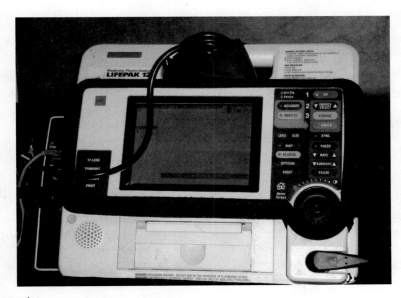

FIGURE 5–10. Cardiac monitor

 KEY POINTS TO REMEMBER

1. An electrode is an adhesive pad that contains conductive gel, is designed to be attached to the patient's skin, and is connected to the monitor or EKG machine by wires called leads.

2. Leads I, II, and III are known as bipolar leads (standard limb leads), which means these leads have one positive electrode and one negative electrode.

3. The left upper arm lead should be placed on the left upper chest, away from the bony prominences.

4. The right upper arm lead should be placed on the right upper chest.

5. The lower-left lead should be placed on the left lower abdomen.

6. If the monitor has a fourth lead, it should be placed on the right lower abdomen.

7. EKG paper is an arrangement of a series of horizontal and vertical lines printed on graph paper that provides a printed record of cardiac electrical activity.

8. Time is measured on the horizontal line of the EKG paper; amplitude, or voltage, is measured on the vertical line.

9. EKG paper is divided into small squares, each of which is 1 mm in height and width and represents a time interval of 0.04 seconds.

10. Darker lines further divide the paper every fifth square, both vertically and horizontally.

11. A wave or waveform recorded on an EKG strip refers to movement away from the baseline or isoelectric line, and is represented as a positive deflection (above the isoelectric line) or as a negative deflection (below the isoelectric line).

12. The P wave represents depolarization of both the left and right atria.

13. The PR interval represents the time interval necessary for the impulse to travel from the SA node, through the internodal pathways in the atria, and downward to the ventricles.

14. The QRS complex represents the conduction of the electrical impulse from the bundle of His throughout the ventricular muscle, or ventricular depolarization.

15. The ST segment is the interval during which the ventricles are depolarized and ventricular repolarization begins. ↳ constriction

16. The T wave represents ventricular repolarization.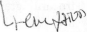

REVIEW QUESTIONS

1. Ventricular diastole refers to ventricular:
  a. Contraction
  b. Relaxation
  c. Filling time
  d. Pressure ratio

2. The electrocardiogram is used to:
  a. Determine cardiac output
  b. Detect valvular dysfunction
  c. Evaluate electrical activity in the heart
  d. Detect left-to-right conduction disorders

3. The PR interval should normally be _0.12 to 0.20_ seconds or smaller.
  a. 0.10   **c.** 0.08
  b. 0.12   **d.** 0.20

4. The QRS interval should normally be _____ seconds or smaller.
  a. 0.20   **c.** 0.18
  b. 0.12   **d.** 0.36

5. The QRS complex is produced when:
  a. The ventricles repolarize
  b. The ventricles depolarize
  c. The ventricles contract
  d. Both b and c

6. The normal conduction pattern of the heart follows which sequence?
  1. SA node
  2. Purkinje fibers 6
  3. Bundle of His 4
  4. AV node 3

5. Bundle branches 5
6. Internodal pathways ✓
  a. 1, 5, 2, 4, 6, 3
  b. 1, 6, 4, 3, 5, 2
  c. 1, 4, 3, 6, 5, 2
  d. 1, 2, 3, 4, 5, 6

7. The T wave on the EKG strip represents:
  a. Rest period
  b. Bundle of His
  c. Atrial contraction
  d. Ventricular contraction

8. The coronary circulation has how many main arteries?
  a. Two L & R   **c.** Four
  b. Six   **d.** Eight

9. When interpreting dysrhythmias, the health care provider should remember that the most important key is the:
  a. PR interval
  b. Rate and rhythm
  c. Presence of dysrhythmias
  d. Patient's clinical appearance

10. A graphic record of the electrical activity of the heart is an:
  a. Echocardiogram   **c.** Encephalogram
  b. Electrocardiogram   **d.** Radiogram

11. While EKG analysis serves as a useful diagnostic tool, the health care professional must be cognizant of the fact that the EKG is a graphic tracing of the electrical activity of the heart but not the mechanical activity.

a. True   b. False

12. The ground lead serves to minimize outside electrical interference.

a. True   b. False

13. The exact portion of the heart being visualized depends, in large part, on the placement of the:

a. Patient   c. Electrodes
b. Paddles   d. Oscilloscope

14. Lead II is most commonly used for cardiac monitoring because of its ability to visualize _____ waves.

a. P   c. R
b. Q   d. T

15. _____ leads are those that have one positive electrode and one negative electrode.

a. Bipolar   c. Multipolar
b. Unipolar   d. Tripolar

Objectives

Upon completion of this chapter, the student will be able to:

- Recall the general rules to use when correctly identifying heart rhythms
- Describe the basic approach to interpretation of EKG strips
- Discuss the five steps used in interpretation of EKG strips
- Explain how to calculate heart rate, given a 6-second strip
- Name four causes of artifact

Interpretation of an EKG Strip

INTRODUCTION

This is the most important chapter in this textbook! Why would I make such an emphatic statement? Simply because it's true. The preceding chapters were essential building blocks leading up to this chapter, and the subsequent chapters focus on application of the rules mastered in this chapter. Therefore, this chapter is critical to your understanding of proper interpretation of an EKG rhythm strip. For many years now, I have explained to students that the key to learning, interpreting, and—most importantly—*understanding* dysrhythmias is a systematic approach, which must be used each and every time a strip is analyzed.

Now, let's be honest here. Do I really expect you to believe that all paramedics/health care professionals—even the ones who have been "street medics/health care professionals" for 20 years—always apply this five-step systematic approach for every strip they see? Well, no, not exactly. However, you are utilizing this book because you wish to learn how to interpret dysrhythmias effortlessly. Keep in mind that, while learning this skill, memorization will *not* suffice. You must learn and apply this systematic approach to EKG analysis. When you look at a strip, think about and apply these five steps, and you should be successful in mastering the art of EKG analysis.

GENERAL RULES

Here are a few basic rules that will assist you in your quest to correctly identify heart rhythms.

1. **First, and most important, look at your patient!** What is the patient's clinical picture, and how is it significant to the rhythm noted on the monitor?
2. Read EVERY strip from left to right, starting at the beginning of the strip.
3. Apply the five-step systematic approach that you will learn in this chapter.
4. Avoid shortcuts and assumptions. A quick glance at a strip will often lead to an incorrect interpretation.
5. Ask and answer each question in the five-step approach in the order that it is presented here. This is important for consistency.
6. You must master the accepted limits, or parameters, for each dysrhythmia and then apply them to each of the five steps when analyzing the strip.

THE FIVE-STEP APPROACH

There are several appropriate formats for EKG interpretation. The format that I have chosen follows a logical sequence in that we discuss EKG interpretation first on the basis of heart rate and rhythm and then by analysis of graphic representations of activities as they occur in the electrical conduction system of the heart.

This five-step approach, in order of application, includes analysis of the following:

1. **Step 1**: Heart rate
2. **Step 2**: Heart rhythm
3. **Step 3**: P wave
4. **Step 4**: PR interval
5. **Step 5**: QRS complex

EKG interpretation is more easily mastered if each step is examined using this approach with each strip. Remember: A quick glance can be deceiving, so do not take a chance.

Step 1: Heart rate

Heart rate can be defined as the number of electrical impulses (as represented by PQRST complexes) conducted through the myocardium in 60 seconds (1 min). This analysis should be your first step in the interpretation of an EKG strip. When calculating heart rate, we are usually referring to the **ventricular** heart rate. However, it is appropriate in certain strips to calculate both the atrial heart rate and the ventricular heart rate.

Simply stated, atrial heart rate can be determined by counting the number of P waves noted; ventricular heart rate is determined by counting the number of QRS complexes. If the atrial and ventricular heart rates are dissimilar, it is very important that you calculate both.

Recall now that the sinoatrial (SA) node discharges impulses at a rate of 60 to 100 times per minute. Therefore, a "normal" heart rate will be noted if the rate is calculated within a range of 60 to 100 beats per minute (BPM). If the rate is noted to be less than 60 BPM, we refer to it as **bradycardia**. In contrast, if the heart rate is greater than 100 BPM, the correct term is **tachycardia**. It is important to note here that these numbers are simply normal boundaries (sometimes called parameters) to which we adhere when analyzing heart rate.

Keep in mind that your patient's clinical picture is critical to proper assessment and management. In other words, if your patient's heart rate is 58 BPM, he or she is *technically* bradycardic, on the basis of "normal" parameters. The patient's clinical picture, however, may indicate no evidence of compromise. Remember to ask yourself this question: **How is the rhythm significant to the patient's clinical picture?** Often you will find that the patient with a heart rate of 58 BPM is exhibiting no clinical symptomatology at all.

There are two methods commonly used to determine heart rate by visual examination of an EKG strip. The first and simplest is called the 6-second method. (See ■ **Figure 6–1**.) To use this method properly you must first denote a 6-second interval on an EKG strip. Fortunately for us, EKG paper is commonly marked in either 3- or 6-second increments. Simply count the number of QRS complexes that occur within the 6-second interval and then multiply this number by 10. If the graph paper does not have 3- or 6-second marks, you can count the number of R waves in 30 large squares and multiply this number by 10. This will yield a close approximation of the patient's heart rate. This method is effective even when the rhythm is noted to be irregular.

The second common method used to determine heart rate by visual examination of an EKG strip is the *R-R interval* method. This method is most accurate if the heart rhythm is regular; otherwise, it is only an estimation of heart rate. Recall from our discussion of EKG graph paper that there are 300 large boxes in a 60-second, or 1-minute, strip. With this in mind, you should look for a QRS complex (specifically an R wave) that falls on a

heart rate the number of electrical impulses conducted through the myocardium in 60 seconds

bradycardia heart rate of less than 60 BPM

tachycardia heart rate greater than 100 BPM

8 complexes in 6 seconds approximates to 80/min (8 × 10 = 80)

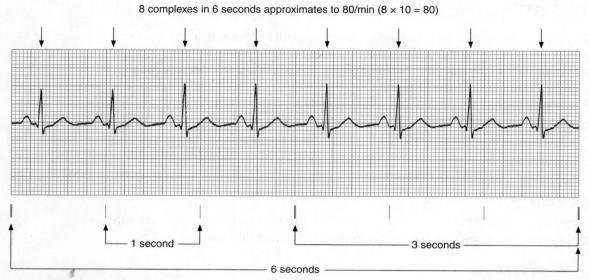

FIGURE 6–1. The 6-second method

heavy line on the strip. Then you should count the number of large boxes between the first R wave and the next R wave. After you determine that number, you divide it into 300. For example, if there are three large boxes between two R-to-R waves, you would divide 3 into 300 and find that the heart rate is 100 BPM (300 ÷ 3 = 100). Apply this method to the strip in ■ **Figure 6–2**.

Remember that the "normal" heart rate is 60 to 100 BPM. Below 60 BPM is a slow, or bradycardic, rate. Greater than 100 BPM is considered a fast, or tachycardic, rate. Heart rates can vary depending on many factors, including the general health of your patient, as well as stress levels, strenuous exercise, or myocardial compromise. Again, you must constantly assess your patient's clinical picture while assessing his or her EKG strip.

Step 2: Heart rhythm

Now we are ready to move on to step 2 in the systematic approach to EKG analysis. Step 2 involves evaluating the rhythm of the heart. The term **heart rhythm** can be defined as the sequential beating of the heart as a result of the generation of electrical impulses. Synonyms for rhythm include pattern, guide, model, order, and design. Thus, we can see that calculating the heart rhythm involves establishing a pattern of QRS complex occurrence. Calculations of heart rhythms are classified as either regular or irregular.

heart rhythm the sequential beating of the heart as a result of the generation of electrical impulses

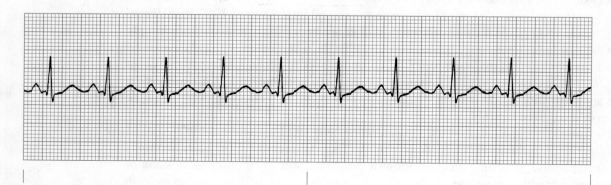

FIGURE 6–2. NSR strip with rate of 100

Normally, the heart's rhythm is regular. To determine whether the ventricular rhythm is regular, you should measure the intervals between R to R waves. To determine whether the atrial rhythm is regular, you should measure the intervals between P to P waves. We can consider the rhythm regular if the intervals vary by less than 0.06 seconds (or 1.5 small squares). If, however, the intervals are variable by greater than 0.06 seconds, the rhythm is considered irregular.

one or more small box

It may be helpful to use EKG calipers when you begin to analyze EKG rhythms. If calipers are not available, you may also measure intervals by making marks on a piece of paper placed on the EKG strip just below the peak of the R wave. After marking the area where each R wave occurred, look at the marks on your paper to identify a pattern. Then, measure the distance between the marks with a ruler. If the marks are relatively equal distances apart, the rhythm is noted to be regular. If the distance between the marks varies noticeably, then the rhythm is probably irregular. Alterations of respiratory rate and depth may produce slight variations in heart rhythms.

Rhythms that are found to be irregular can be further classified as:

a. *Regularly irregular*—irregular rhythms that occur in a pattern.
b. *Occasionally irregular*—intervals of only one or two R-Rs are uneven.
c. *Irregularly irregular*—R-R intervals exhibit no similarity.

Regardless of whether the rhythm is regular or irregular, always remember to ask yourself the all-important question: **How is this rhythm clinically significant to my patient?**

Before moving on to step 3, take a moment to review steps 1 and 2. Now look at the two strips in ■ **Figures 6–3 and 6–4** and calculate the rate and rhythm of each one. After you think you have the answers, ask your instructor or tutor to verify your answers.

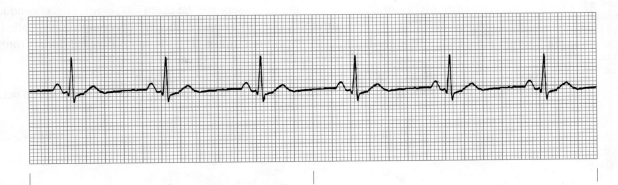

FIGURE 6–3. Practice strips for rate and rhythm analysis

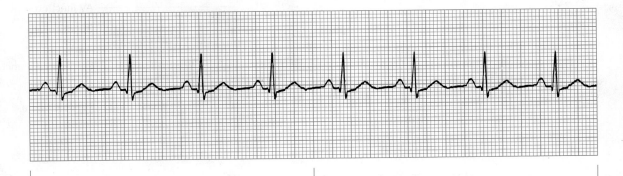

FIGURE 6–4. Practice strips for rate and rhythm analysis

Step 3: The P wave

First, let's recall the events that must occur to cause the formation of P waves on an EKG strip. We learned in Chapter 5 that the P wave is produced when the right and left atria depolarize. Depolarization of the atria is produced when an electrical impulse spreads throughout the atria via the internodal pathways. The P wave is noted as the first deviation from the isoelectric line on the EKG strip and should always be rounded and upright (positive) in chest Lead II. If the P wave is not upright in Lead II, you are not looking at a sinus rhythm (i.e., a rhythm originating in the SA node).

There are five questions that should be asked in evaluating P waves:

1. Are P waves present?
2. Are the P waves occurring regularly?
3. Is there one P wave present for each QRS complex present?
4. Are the P waves smooth, rounded, and upright (positive) in appearance, or are they inverted?
5. Do all the P waves look similar?

Recall now that the SA node is the primary pacemaker of the heart and is located in the right atrium (See ■ **Figure 6–5**). If the SA node is pacing or firing at regular intervals, the P waves will also follow at regular intervals. This pattern would then be referred to as a **sinus rhythm**. In this text, the heart rhythms will be referred to according to their points of origin.

Step 4: The PR interval

PR interval
measures the time intervals from the onset of atrial contraction to the onset of ventricular contraction

The **PR interval** measures the time intervals from the onset of atrial contraction to the onset of ventricular contraction, or the time necessary for the electrical impulse to be conducted through the atria and the atrioventricular (AV) node. Although this component is called the PR interval, it actually includes the entire P wave. The PR interval is measured from the onset (beginning) of the P wave to the onset of the Q wave of the QRS complex.

The normal length of the PR interval is 0.12 to 0.20 seconds (3–5 small squares). The PR interval should be constant across the EKG strip in order to be considered "within normal

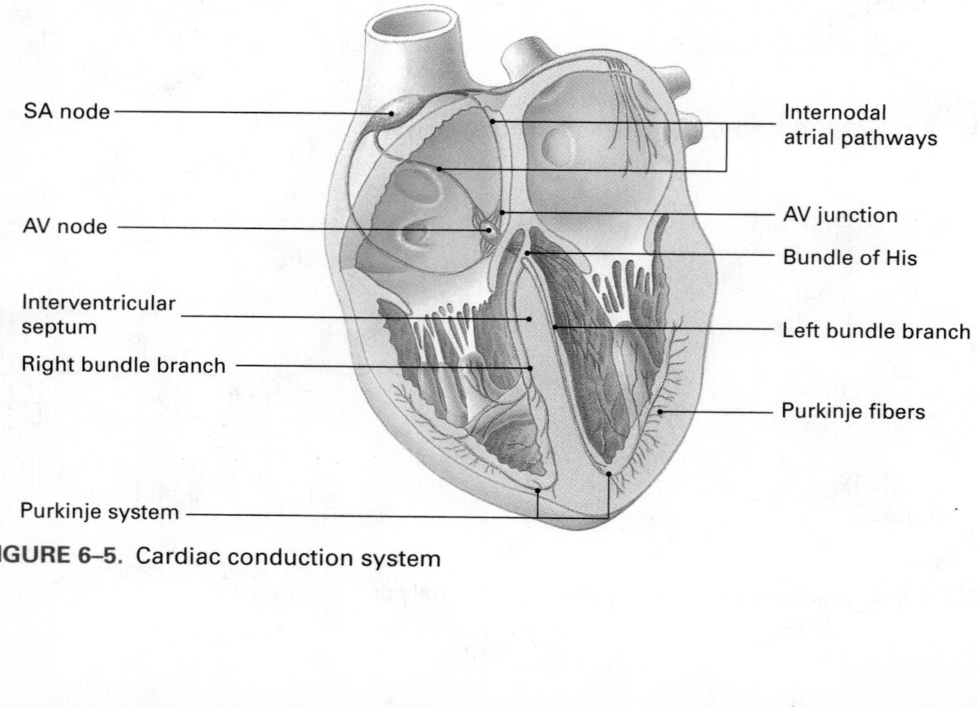

SA node

Internodal atrial pathways

AV node

AV junction

Bundle of His

Interventricular septum

Left bundle branch

Right bundle branch

Purkinje fibers

Purkinje system

FIGURE 6–5. Cardiac conduction system

limits." A shortened PR interval (less than 0.12 sec) may be an indication that the usual progression of the impulse was outside the normal route. Prolonged PR intervals (greater than 0.20 sec) may indicate a delay in the electrical conduction pathway or an AV block.

There are three questions that should be asked when evaluating PR intervals:

1. Are PR intervals greater than 0.20 seconds?
2. Are PR intervals less than 0.12 seconds?
3. Are PR intervals constant across the EKG strip?

Step 5: The QRS complex

The **QRS complex** represents the depolarization (or contraction) of the ventricles. It is important to note whether all QRS complexes look alike, as this similarity will indicate that conduction pathways are invariable and consistent.

The QRS complex is actually a group of waves, consisting of:

Q wave—the first negative or downward deflection of this large complex. It is a small wave that precedes the R wave. Often, the Q wave is not seen.

R wave—the first upward or positive deflection following the P wave. In chest Lead II, the R wave is the tallest waveform noted.

S wave—the sharp, negative (or downward) deflection that follows the R wave.

The overall appearance of the QRS, as well as its width, can provide important information about the electrical conduction system. When the electrical conduction system is functioning normally, the width of the QRS complex will be 0.12 seconds or less (narrow). This normal, or narrow, QRS complex indicates that the impulse was not formed in the ventricles and is thus referred to as **supraventricular**, "above the ventricles." Wide QRS complexes (greater than 0.12 sec or 3 small squares) indicate that the impulse is either of ventricular origin or of supraventricular origin with conduction that is aberrant (deviating from the normal course or pattern).

There are three questions that should be asked in evaluating QRS intervals:

1. Are QRS intervals greater than 0.12 seconds (wide)? If so, the complex may be ventricular in origin.
2. Are QRS intervals less than 0.12 seconds (narrow)? If so, the complex is probably supraventricular in origin.
3. Are the QRS complexes similar in appearance across the EKG strip?

It is important to realize that the shape of QRS complexes will vary slightly in individual patients, depending on factors such as heart shape and size, health of the myocardium, and location and placement of electrodes.

ST SEGMENT

The **ST segment** begins with the end of the QRS complex and ends with the onset of the T wave. The normal ST segment is usually consistent with the isoelectric line of the EKG strip. The point where the QRS complex meets the ST segment is commonly referred to as the **J point**. (See ■ **Figure 6–6**.) If the ST segment is depressed, myocardial ischemia may be indicated. If the ST segment is elevated, it would be indicative of acute myocardial injury. The ramifications of ST segment elevation and depression are discussed in detail in the companion book to this text, *Understanding 12-Lead EKGs: A Practical Approach,* 3rd Edition.

QRS complex represents the depolarization (or contraction) of the ventricles

supraventricular above the ventricles

ST segment begins with the end of the QRS complex and ends with the onset of the T wave

J point the point where the QRS complex meets the ST segment

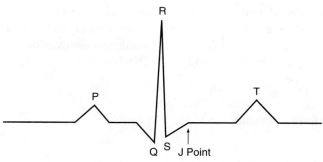

FIGURE 6–6. J point

THE T WAVE

T wave produced by ventricular repolarization or relaxation

The **T wave** is produced by ventricular repolarization or relaxation. Recall our discussion of the heart's refractory periods (see Chapter 3) to emphasize the importance of the T wave. T waves are commonly seen as the first upward or positive deflection following the QRS complex.

THE U WAVE

U waves are usually not visible on EKG strips, and their cause or origin is not completely understood. Some cardiovascular physiologists now believe that the U wave may represent Purkinje fiber repolarization. It is also theorized that U-waves may be caused by medications such as amiodarone, digoxin, procainamide, and others. When they can be distinguished, U waves typically follow the T wave. The U wave, when present, will appear much smaller than the T wave and will commonly be rounded and upright or positive in deflection.

ARTIFACT

artifact EKG waveforms from sources outside the heart

Artifact is defined as EKG waveforms from sources outside the heart. Artifact is interference seen on a monitor or an EKG strip. (See ■ **Figure 6–7.**) Following are four common causes of artifact:

1. **Patient movement**—One type of artifact, called a wandering baseline, may be produced when the patient moves about on the bed or gurney and can usually be corrected when the patient lies still.

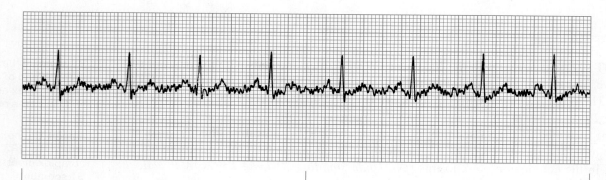

FIGURE 6–7. Artifact

2. **Loose or defective electrodes**—When electrodes have lost contact with the patient's skin or when the conductive gel on the electrode has dried, one type of artifact—which may appear as a "fuzzy baseline"—is called 60-cycle interference. This may also result from clammy skin or excessive chest hair. Interference from electrical equipment may also cause 60-cycle interference.

3. **Improper grounding**—Artifact can occur when the patient is in touch with an outside source of electricity, such as a poorly grounded electrical bed; 60-cycle interference may also be caused by improper grounding.

4. **Faulty EKG apparatus**—Broken wires or cables may produce artifact. This is easily corrected by replacing the faulty wires with new ones.

Artifacts can mimic certain lethal dysrhythmias. Therefore, ongoing **patient assessment is critical.** Remember that if your patient is lying quietly on the gurney or bed and is engaging in a lively conversation with you regarding his or her past medical history, chances are very good that he or she is not in ventricular fibrillation, regardless of what the monitor shows!

CHAPTER 6

 ## SUMMARY

This is the most important chapter in this textbook, in that you must have a logical, systematic approach to interpreting EKGs. It is imperative that you follow this approach each time you practice EKG analysis, both to increase your confidence as well as to ensure accuracy in interpretation and, consequently, in your provision of patient care.

 ## KEY POINTS TO REMEMBER

1. Look at your patient's condition.
2. Read every strip from left to right.
3. Apply the five-step approach.
4. Avoid shortcuts; ask and answer each step in the five-step approach.
5. Heart rate is defined as the number of electrical complexes conducted through the myocardium in 60 seconds.
6. Heart rhythm is defined as the sequential beating of the heart as a result of the generation of electrical impulses.
7. The P wave is produced when the right and left atria depolarize.
8. The PR interval measures the time interval from the onset of atrial contraction to the onset of ventricular contraction.
9. The QRS complex represents the depolarization of the ventricles.
10. The T wave is produced by ventricular repolarization or relaxation.

REVIEW QUESTIONS

1. When dealing with EKG interpretation, you should always avoid shortcuts and assumptions because often a quick glance at a strip will lead to an incorrect interpretation.
   a. False   b. True

2. The intrinsic firing rate of the AV node is _____ BPM.
   a. 15–25   c. 35–45
   b. 25–35   d. 40–60

3. You must master the accepted parameters for each dysrhythmia and then apply those parameters to each of the five steps when analyzing an EKG strip.
   a. True   b. False

4. The electrocardiogram is used to:
   a. Determine pulse rate
   b. Detect valvular dysfunction
   c. Evaluate electrical activity in the heart
   d. Determine whether the heart is beating

5. The PR interval should normally be _____ seconds or smaller.
   a. 0.10   c. 0.08
   b. 0.12   d. 0.20

6. The QRS interval should normally be _____ seconds or smaller.
   a. 0.20   c. 0.18
   b. 0.12   d. 0.36

7. Artifact is defined as EKG waveforms from sources outside the heart.
   a. True   b. False

8. Causes of artifact include:
   a. Patient movement   c. Improper grounding
   b. Loose electrodes   d. All the above apply

9. The point at which the QRS complex meets the ST segment is commonly referred to as the:
   a. T point   c. PRI
   b. J point   d. S point

10. The term supraventricular refers to a stimulus arising above the ventricles.
    a. True   b. False

11. The T wave on the EKG strip represents:
    a. Rest period
    b. Bundle of His
    c. Atrial contraction
    d. Ventricular contraction

12. When interpreting dysrhythmias, you should remember that the most important key is the:
    a. PR interval
    b. Rate and rhythm
    c. Presence of dysrhythmias
    d. Patient's clinical appearance

13. The health care professional should read EVERY EKG strip from left to right, starting at the beginning of the strip.
    a. True   b. False

14. The sharp, negative deflection that follows the R wave is called the Q wave.
    a. True   b. False

15. Heart rhythms are classified as either regular or irregular.
    a. True   b. False

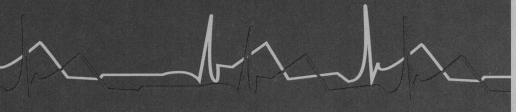

Introducing the Sinus Rhythms

Objectives

Upon completion of this chapter, the student will be able to:

- Explain the origin of the sinus rhythms
- Identify the components of the electrical conduction system of the heart
- Recall the primary pacemakers in the heart and name the intrinsic firing rate of each
- Identify a normal sinus rhythm, including EKG characteristics
- Describe a sinus bradycardia rhythm, including EKG characteristics
- Identify a sinus tachycardia rhythm, including EKG characteristics
- Describe a sinus dysrhythmia, including EKG characteristics
- Describe a sinus arrest rhythm, including EKG characteristics
- Discuss the clinical significance of the sinus rhythms

INTRODUCTION

The time has now come for you to begin to apply the knowledge that you gained from studying Chapters 1–6. You learned in Chapter 6 that you must always, always apply the five-step approach to each rhythm strip as you attempt to interpret the rhythm. For the sake of emphasis, let's call this the golden rule of EKG interpretation: No shortcuts are allowed!

You will ask yourself five essential questions, and when you decide on the answer to each question, you will be able to interpret the rhythm. When you find one parameter that falls out of the normal range, it should raise a "red flag" in your thought processes. The "red flag" method works very well, especially for the novice student. Remember that any abnormal heart rhythm is most commonly referred to as a *dysrhythmia*.

In this and subsequent chapters, you will be interpreting strips from actual patients as well as strips produced from EKG simulators. Remember that rhythm presentations will vary from patient to patient; regardless of the appearance of the waveforms, it is essential that you ask the five questions you have mastered. Only then will you be able to decide which rhythm you are observing. Don't be afraid to ask for help. It takes time and practice to master the art of EKG interpretation.

ORIGIN OF THE SINUS RHYTHMS

As we begin to examine heart rhythms, it is important to remember that rhythms are classified according to the heart structure or structures in which they begin—in other words, their **site of origin**. It is also helpful to think about the *name* of each rhythm in order to recall the site of origin of that specific rhythm. Recall now that the sinoatrial (SA) node normally generates impulses at a rate of 60 to 100 beats per minute (BPM). This characteristic is known as the inherent, or intrinsic, rate of the heart's primary pacemaker, the SA node. Thus, rhythms that originate in the SA node are called either sinus rhythms or sinus dysrhythmias.

site of origin rhythms are classified according to the heart structure or structures in which they begin

COMPONENTS OF THE ELECTRICAL CONDUCTION SYSTEM OF THE HEART

Let's review briefly the components of the electrical conduction system. Normally, the electrical impulse originates in the SA node, which is located in the upper right atrium. As the impulse leaves the SA node, it travels through the atria via the internodal pathways. The impulse then reaches the atrioventricular (AV) node, where there is a brief pause. We often consider the AV node the "gatekeeper" to the ventricles. Leaving the AV node, the electrical impulse travels through the right and left bundle branches into and through the Purkinje fibers of the ventricular musculature.

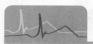

TABLE 7–1 Electrical conduction system pathway

SA node	Internodal pathways	AV node	Bundle of His	Bundle branches	Purkinje network

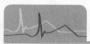

TABLE 7–2 Pacemaker sites

SA (sinoatrial) node	Intrinsic rate of 60–100 BPM
AV (atrioventricular) node	Intrinsic rate of 40–60 BPM
Purkinje network	Intrinsic rate of 20–40 BPM

Included in the heart's electrical conduction system are three pacemaker sites—the SA node, the AV node, and the Purkinje network. The SA node is the primary pacemaker; the AV node and the Purkinje network are the backup, or secondary, pacemakers. The SA node is located in the upper right atrium and has an inherent firing rate of 60 to 100 BPM. The AV node is located on the floor of the right atrium and has an intrinsic firing rate of 40 to 60 BPM. The Purkinje fibers are located in the septum and in the ventricles and have an intrinsic firing rate of 20 to 40 BPM. On the basis of your knowledge of the intrinsic firing rate of the SA node, what would you expect the rate of a sinus rhythm to be? By this time you may have immediately thought: 60 to 100 BPM! If so, you're on your way. Remember that the first question to ask yourself in the five-step approach is: What is the heart rate? Now, let's review once more. (See ■ **Tables 7–1** and **7–2**.)

NORMAL SINUS RHYTHM

normal sinus rhythm the rhythm that occurs when the SA node has generated an impulse that followed the normal pathway of the electrical conduction system and led to atrial and ventricular depolarization

In reality, the *only* "normal" rhythm is normal sinus rhythm (NSR). When you ask the questions in the five-step approach, the answers you derive will be, and must be, within normal limits in order for you to acknowledge that the rhythm you are analyzing is indeed a **normal sinus rhythm**. Although the appearance of the waves can vary, if the answers to all five questions are within normal limits, the rhythm is, quite simply, normal. The SA node has generated an impulse that followed the normal pathway of the electrical conduction system and led to atrial and ventricular depolarization.

The heart rate falls within the range of 60 to 100 BPM, the atrial and ventricular rhythms are regular (a variation of 10% is acceptable), there is a P wave that preceded every QRS complex, all PR intervals (PRIs) range from 0.12 to 0.20 seconds in length, and the QRS complex is less than 0.12 seconds. In other words, all five parameters are within normal limits. The rhythm is a normal sinus rhythm. (See ■ **Table 7–3**.)

Now you should look at the rhythm in ■ **Figure 7–1** and slowly, systematically apply each of the five questions, in order to *prove* to yourself that this rhythm is indeed a normal sinus rhythm. In Figure 7–1, you should find the following parameters:

- Rate = 70 BPM
- Rhythm = Regular
- P wave = Present and upright
- PR Interval = 0.16 sec
- QRS Complex = 0.06 sec

As you should have just proven to yourself, Figure 7–1 represents a Normal Sinus Rhythm! **Remember . . . always monitor your patient's clinical condition!**

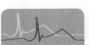

3/25/16

TABLE 7–3 Normal sinus rhythm

Questions 1–5	Answers
1. What is the rate?	60–100 BPM
2. What is the rhythm?	Atrial rhythm regular
	Ventricular rhythm regular
3. Is there a P wave before each QRS?	Yes
Are the P waves upright and uniform?	Yes
4. What is the length of the PR interval?	0.12–0.20 sec (3–5 small squares)
5. Do all the QRS complexes look alike?	Yes
What is the Length of the QRS Complexes?	Less than 0.12 sec (3 small squares)

ST Segmen
T wave

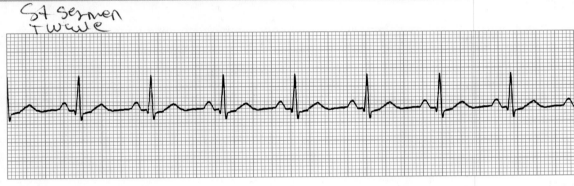

FIGURE 7–1. Normal sinus rhythm

SINUS BRADYCARDIA RHYTHM

In initial lectures (and just for fun), I often tell students that a normal sinus rhythm has two "first cousins," sinus bradycardia and sinus tachycardia. One of those cousins will be discussed here now, the other next. At first glance, this rhythm may resemble a normal sinus rhythm, and as a matter of fact the only difference between sinus bradycardia rhythm and normal sinus rhythm is the heart rate. Because of this one variable, however, this sinus bradycardia rhythm is *not* normal.

Sinus bradycardia is often called sinus brady. Recall from your knowledge of medical terminology, that the term *brady* means slow. In this rhythm, the SA node discharges impulses at a rate of less than 60 BPM.

Sinus bradycardia may be caused by intrinsic disease of the SA node, vomiting, electrolyte imbalances, hypoxia, hypothermia, or the effects of certain drugs, such as morphine, digitalis, beta blockers, calcium channel blockers, and some sedatives. Do we panic when we note a sinus bradycardia on a rhythm strip? No, we don't panic over *any* rhythm. We simply consider the ramifications of that rhythm, based on our patient's clinical condition. As a matter of fact, in a person who is sleeping and in a young, well-conditioned athlete, we expect to see some degree of sinus bradycardia as a normal phenomenon. Later in this chapter, we will discuss the clinical significance of this rhythm and other sinus dysrhythmias.

Now, let's apply our five-step approach to analyzing this rhythm. (See ■ **Table 7–4** and ■ **Figure 7–2**.) You should note the heart rate as 40 BPM, the rhythm is regular, P wave is

sinus bradycardia
in this rhythm, the SA node discharges impulses at a rate of less than 60 BPM

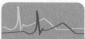

TABLE 7–4 Sinus bradycardia rhythm

Questions 1–5	Answers
1. What is the rate?	Less than 60 BPM
2. What is the rhythm?	Atrial rhythm regular
	Ventricular rhythm regular
3. Is there a P wave before each QRS?	Yes
Are the P waves upright and uniform?	Yes
4. What is the length of the PR interval?	0.12–0.20 sec (3–5 small squares)
5. Do all the QRS complexes look alike?	Yes
What is the length of the QRS complexes?	Less than 0.12 sec (3 small squares)

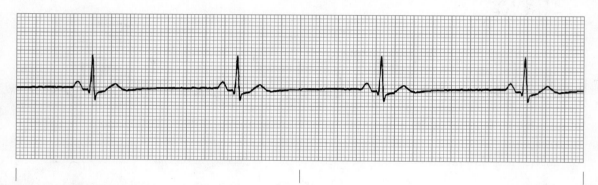

FIGURE 7–2. Sinus bradycardia rhythm

present and upright, the PRI is 0.16 seconds, and the QRS is 0.06 seconds. These findings should validate Sinus Bradycardia.

Remember that sinus bradycardia looks very much like normal sinus rhythm, but the rate is slower (less than 60 BPM). **Remember . . . always monitor your patient's clinical condition.**

SINUS TACHYCARDIA RHYTHM

Sinus tachycardia is the other first cousin of NSR. Tachycardia technically means a fast heart rate, and the term sinus tells us that this rhythm originated in the SA node. Thus we can conclude that **sinus tachycardia** is a variant of normal sinus rhythm, the only difference being the rate of the impulses generated by the SA node. The rate of sinus tachycardia, or sinus tach, is generally considered to be 100 to 160 BPM.

The impulses generated in this rhythm follow the normal pathway of the electrical conduction system. Thus P waves will be present before QRS complexes, the PR interval will be within normal limits, and the QRS complexes will all look similar and will be less than 0.12 seconds in length. The atrial and ventricular rhythms will be regular. As the heart rate approaches the upper limits of the normal range, the P waves may be slightly harder to discern, but they can usually be observed and analyzed.

Causes of sinus tachycardia are numerous, including exercise, fear, stress, pain, anxiety, and ingestion of stimulants such as coffee or alcohol, all of which result in stimulation of the

sinus tachycardia a variant of normal sinus rhythm; the rate is generally considered to be 100 to 160 BPM

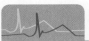

TABLE 7–5 Sinus tachycardia rhythm

Questions 1–5	Answers
1. What is the rate?	100–160 BPM
2. What is the rhythm?	Atrial rhythm regular
	Ventricular rhythm regular
3. Is there a P wave before each QRS?	Yes
Are the P waves upright and uniform?	Yes
4. What is the length of the PR interval?	0.12–0.20 sec (3–5 small squares)
5. Do all the QRS complexes look alike?	Yes
What is the length of the QRS complexes?	Less than 0.12 sec (3 small squares)

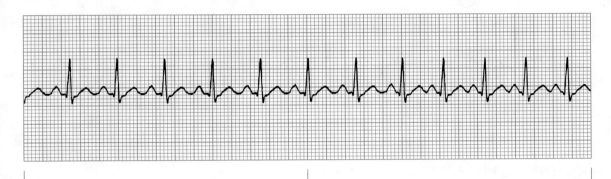

FIGURE 7–3. Sinus tachycardia rhythm

sympathetic nervous system. In addition, sinus tachycardia may result from hypovolemia, congestive heart failure, severe dehydration, or acute myocardial infarction. While it is generally held that sinus tachycardia, in and of itself, is not dangerous to the patient, we should remember that the underlying cause of this rhythm may be quite serious. If the very fast rate decreases the ability of the heart to refill properly, the patient's cardiac output may be reduced. In this instance it becomes very important that the underlying cause of the rhythm be identified and corrected as soon as possible. Remember that the KEY to properly identifying this rhythm is the *heart rate*.

Again, we apply our five-step approach to analyzing this rhythm. (See ■ **Table 7–5** and ■ **Figure 7–3**.)

You should note the heart rate as 120 BPM, the rhythm is regular, P wave is present and upright, the PRI is 0.16 seconds, and the QRS is 0.04 seconds. These findings should validate Sinus Tachycardia.

Remember that sinus tachycardia looks very much like normal sinus rhythm, but the rate is faster (more than 100 BPM). **Remember . . . always monitor your patient's clinical condition**.

SINUS DYSRHYTHMIA

Sinus dysrhythmia resembles other sinus rhythms, except for the slight irregularity of the heart rhythm. The rate of impulse formation in the SA node may vary with respirations. In this rhythm, impulses are initiated by the SA node but at irregular intervals. An irregular

sinus dysrhythmia
an irregular rhythm produced when the P-to-P intervals and the R-to-R intervals change with respirations

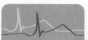

TABLE 7–6 Sinus dysrhythmia

Questions 1–5	Answers
1. What is the rate?	60–100 BPM
2. What is the rhythm?	Irregular (variance of more than 0.08 sec)
3. Is there a P wave before each QRS?	Yes
Are the P waves upright and uniform?	Yes
4. What is the length of the PR interval?	0.12–0.20 sec (3–5 small squares)
5. Do all the QRS complexes look alike?	Yes
What is the length of the QRS complexes?	Less than 0.12 sec (3 small squares)

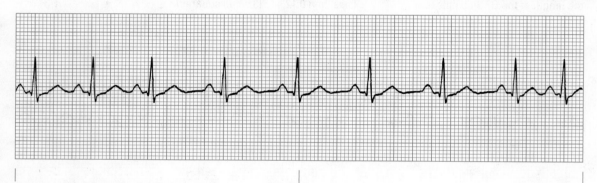

FIGURE 7–4. Sinus dysrhythmia rhythm

rhythm is produced when the P-to-P intervals and the R-to-R intervals change with respirations. In Sinus Dysrhythmia, the heart rate increases during inspiration and decreases during expiration, related to changes in intrathoracic pressure. As a general rule, there should be a difference of at least 0.08 seconds between the shortest and longest R-R intervals in order to determine that the rhythm is not a normal sinus rhythm. A very careful step-by-step approach is necessary to distinguish sinus dysrhythmia.

Sinus dysrhythmia is a common and normal finding, especially in children and young adults. Causes of sinus dysrhythmia may include the administration of certain drugs such as digitalis, underlying cardiac disease such as sick sinus syndrome, or myocardial infarction. Remember that the KEY to identifying this rhythm properly is the *heart rhythm*. Again, we apply our five-step approach to analyzing this rhythm. (See ■ **Table 7–6** and ■ **Figure 7–4**.)

You should note the heart rate as 90 BPM, the rhythm is irregular, P wave is present and upright, the PRI is 0.16 seconds, and the QRS is 0.04 seconds. These findings should validate Sinus Dysrhythmia.

Remember that sinus dysrhythmia looks very much like normal sinus rhythm, but the rhythm is slightly irregular, varying with respirations. **Remember . . . always monitor your patient's clinical condition.**

SINUS ARREST RHYTHM

sinus arrest rhythm when the sinus node fails to discharge, the absence of a PQRST interval is noted on the rhythm strip

When the SA node fails to initiate an impulse, a rhythm known as **sinus arrest rhythm** results. When the sinus node fails to discharge, the absence of a PQRST interval is noted on the rhythm strip. This occurrence causes a slight period of cardiac standstill, which lasts

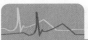

TABLE 7–7 Sinus arrest rhythm

Questions 1–5	Answers
1. What is the rate?	Variable, depending on the frequency of sinus arrest
2. What is the rhythm?	Irregular, when sinus arrest is present
3. Is there a P wave before each QRS?	Yes—if QRS is present
Are the P waves upright and uniform?	Yes—if QRS is present
4. What is the length of the PR interval?	0.12–0.20 sec (3–5 small squares)
5. Do all the QRS complexes look alike?	Yes, when present
What is the length of the QRS complexes?	Less than 0.12 sec (3 small squares)

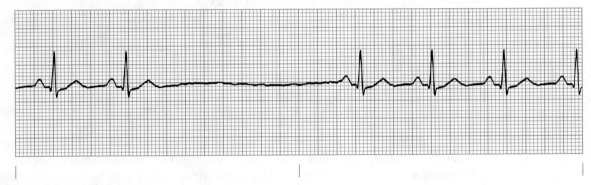

FIGURE 7–5. Sinus arrest rhythm

until the sinus node continues its normal function. The absence of a PQRST complex appears as a pause on the EKG strip. This rhythm can quickly get your attention! However, if these occurrences are infrequent, there may be no immediate cause for undue concern. Patient assessment is imperative.

Causes of sinus arrest may include hypoxia, ischemia, damage to the SA node, or certain drugs, such as digitalis or salicylates. Sinus arrest can also occur as a result of myocardial infarction. Remember that the KEY to properly identifying this rhythm is the **transient absence of the PQRST complexes.** Now, let's apply our five-step approach to analyzing this rhythm. (See ■ **Table 7–7** and ■ **Figure 7–5.**)

You should note the heart rate as 60 BPM, the rhythm is irregular, P wave is present and upright, the PRI is 0.16 seconds, and the QRS is 0.06 seconds. These findings should validate Sinus Arrest.

Remember that sinus arrest presents as an infrequent absence of a PQRST complex. **Remember . . . always monitor your patient's clinical condition.**

CLINICAL SIGNIFICANCE OF SINUS RHYTHMS

The clinical significance of sinus rhythms is directly associated with the assessment of your patient. Often, sinus rhythms are not particularly significant or serious. As with all rhythms, patient assessment is crucial to determining the patient's tolerance of the dysrhythmia. Determine whether your patient is medically stable or medically unstable. If the patient is experiencing chest pains, dizziness, weakness, fainting, markedly decreased or increased blood pressure, or alterations in level of consciousness, he or she is considered symptomatic or medically unstable. We will now discuss the clinical significance of each of the sinus dysrhythmias.

Sinus bradycardia

Recall now that sinus bradycardia is a dysrhythmia commonly seen in young, well-conditioned athletes or in people who are sleeping. However, if the patient's heart rate falls significantly, cardiac compromise will become a cause for concern. If your patient becomes symptomatic, exhibiting signs of decreased cardiac output, treatment should be initiated at once. Treatment for sinus bradycardia may include the administration of oxygen, initiating an IV/IO access line, administering the drug atropine, transcutaneous pacing (TCP), or some combination of these. The use of dopamine IV drip and epinephrine IV drip can also be considered in the treatment of Sinus Bradycardia.

Signs of cardiac compromise may include, but are not limited to, the following: altered mental status, chest pain, hypotension, dizziness, and fainting. Be aware that sinus bradycardia may follow the application of carotid sinus massage (discussed in Chapter 8). When the heart rate becomes extremely slow, ectopic (out-of-place) complexes or rhythms (like PVCs) may occur. Again, look at your patient and evaluate him or her continually.

Sinus tachycardia

Sinus tachycardia usually does not require treatment. Let me be quick to add, however, that it is imperative to seek out and correct the underlying cause of the rapid heart rate. In some cases, sinus tachycardia can be thought of as a double-edged sword. Why is this true? Because, although sinus tachycardia may actually be a compensatory mechanism for decreased stroke volume, it is also true that cardiac output may fall when the heart rate approaches 150 BPM, due to inadequate ventricular filling time. In addition, myocardial oxygen demand increases with rapid heart rates, and this can precipitate myocardial ischemia or even infarct of the myocardial tissue. It should also be noted that sinus tachycardia may result from the administration of drugs, such as epinephrine or from certain stimulants, such as cocaine or excessive amounts of caffeine.

Treatment of sinus tachycardia is aimed at finding and treating the underlying cause. If the patient is hypovolemic, the hypovolemia should be corrected as soon as is feasible. If the patient is complaining of chest pain, oxygen should be administered immediately and the patient should be moved to a definitive care facility. Often, when the underlying cause of this dysrhythmia is identified and managed, the rhythm will gradually convert back to the patient's normal rhythm.

Sinus dysrhythmia

Sinus dysrhythmia is considered a normal alteration in heart rhythm, especially in young children and elderly adults. This rhythm usually does not require emergency intercession.

Sinus arrest

By now, I'm quite sure you have absorbed the idea that all patients, even those with "normal" heart rhythms, must be constantly monitored and assessed. As I mentioned earlier in this chapter, sinus arrest rhythm usually demands our immediate attention, just by virtue of its appearance on the oscilloscope or rhythm strip.

When you begin to analyze a rhythm strip that shows sinus arrest, you (of course) ask the first question: What is the patient's heart rate? As soon as you begin to calculate heart rate, you immediately notice that *something* (namely, a PQRST complex) is missing! Right away, you know that something is wrong, so you look at your patient (yes, again). If the patient appears to be medically stable, you continue with your analysis of the strip.

If your patient is asymptomatic (medically stable) and the episodes of sinus arrest are occurring only occasionally, continued observation may be all that is required. It is prudent to keep in mind that frequent episodes of sinus arrest may cause cardiac compromise. It may be necessary to administer atropine if the patient is bradycardic and exhibits other accompanying symptoms (feelings of faintness or dizziness). If atropine is ineffective, transcutaneous pacing (TCP) may be indicated.

CHAPTER 7

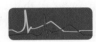 ## SUMMARY

Rhythms that arise from the SA node include normal sinus rhythm, sinus bradycardia, sinus tachycardia, sinus dysrhythmia, and sinus arrest. Common characteristics of the sinus rhythms include the usually normal appearance of P wave morphology, upright P waves in Lead II, and the normal duration of the PR interval and the QRS complex. The only normal rhythm is normal sinus rhythm; all other rhythms in this group are appropriately termed *dysrhythmias*.

 ## KEY POINTS TO REMEMBER

1. Rhythms are classified based on the heart structure in which they begin, or site of origin.
2. The only normal rhythm is normal sinus rhythm, the rate of which is 60 to 100 BPM.
3. Sinus bradycardia resembles NSR; however the rate is slower, that is, 40 to 60 BPM.
4. Sinus tachycardia resembles NSR; however the rate is faster, that is, 100 to 160 BPM.

5. Sinus dysrhythmia resembles other sinus rhythms, except for the slight irregularity of the rhythm.
6. When the SA node fails to initiate an impulse, a sinus arrest will result in a missed complex until the sinus node continues its normal function.
7. Always remember to monitor your patient's clinical condition!

 ## REVIEW QUESTIONS

1. How many chambers are located in the heart?
   a. Five
   b. Three
   c. Four
   d. Six

2. The two upper chambers of the heart are called the:
   a. Ventricles
   b. Atria
   c. Aorta
   d. Vena cava

3. What happens to the blood as it passes through the pulmonary capillaries?
   a. Oxygen is added and carbon dioxide removed.
   b. Carbon dioxide is added and oxygen is removed.
   c. Oxygen is added and carbon dioxide is added.
   d. Oxygen is removed and carbon dioxide is removed.

4. The right ventricle pumps oxygen-poor blood to the lungs through the:
   a. Pulmonary veins   c. Vena cava
   b. Aorta   **d. Pulmonary arteries**

5. What is the normal order of the electrical conduction pattern of the heart?
   a. AV node, SA node, ventricles
   b. Ventricles, AV node, SA node
   c. SA node, ventricles, AV node
   d. SA node, AV node, ventricles

6. An abnormal rhythm of the heart is called a:
   a. Dysrhythmia   c. Rhythmia— *too fast or too slow irregular*
   b. Paranormal rhythm   d. Pararhythm

7. Bradycardia usually refers to a heart rate of _____ BPM.
   a. Less than 70   c. Greater than 60
   b. Less than 60   d. Less than 100

8. Tachycardia usually refers to a heart rate of _____ BPM.
   a. Greater than 100   c. Less than 100
   b. Greater than 80   d. Less than 60

9. The largest artery in the body is the:
   a. Femoral   c. Carotid
   b. Aorta   d. Pulmonary

10. Normal sinus rhythm usually refers to a heart rate of _____ BPM.
    a. Greater than 100
    b. Greater than 110
    c. Less than 100
    d. Between 60 and 100

11. In sinus dysrhythmia, waveforms vary with respirations.
    a. True   b. False   *less than 60*

12. Bradycardia describes a heart rate of less than 70 BPM.
    a. False   b. True

13. If your patient is asymptomatic (medically stable), and episodes of sinus arrest are occurring only occasionally, continued observation may be all that is required.
    a. True   b. False

14. As a general rule, there should be a difference of at least 0.08 seconds between the shortest and longest R-R intervals in order to distinguish that a rhythm is not a normal sinus rhythm.
    a. True   b. False

15. Rhythms that originate in the SA node are called either sinus rhythms or sinus dysrhythmias.
    a. True   b. False

REVIEW STRIPS

1. Rate _____   Rhythm _____
   P wave _____   PR interval _____
   QRS complex _____   Interpretation _____

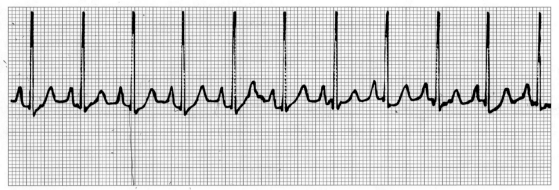

2. Rate _110_ Rhythm _regular_
   P wave _yes_ PR interval _.12 to .20_
   QRS complex _3 box < .12_ Interpretation _Sinus ticycardia_

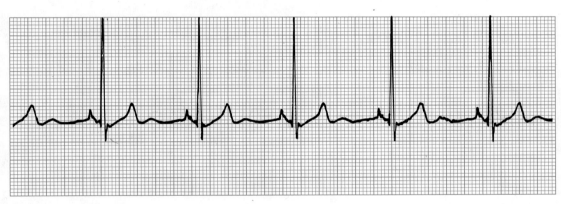

3. Rate _50_ Rhythm _regular_
   P wave _yes_ PR interval _.12 to 20_
   QRS complex _< .12_ Interpretation _Sinus bradycardia_

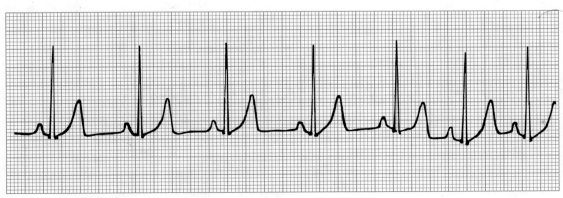

4. Rate _____ Rhythm _____
   P wave _____ PR interval _____
   QRS complex _____ Interpretation _____

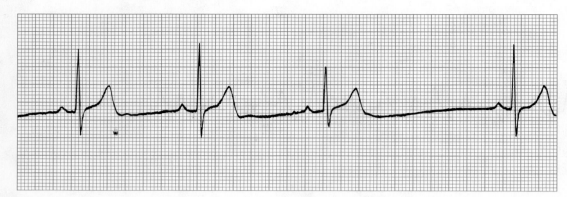

5. Rate _____   Rhythm _____

   P wave _____   PR interval _____

   QRS complex _____   Interpretation _____

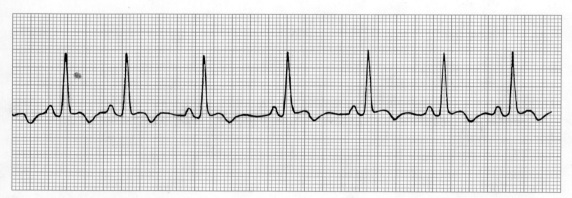

6. Rate _____   Rhythm _____

   P wave _____   PR interval _____

   QRS complex _____   Interpretation _____

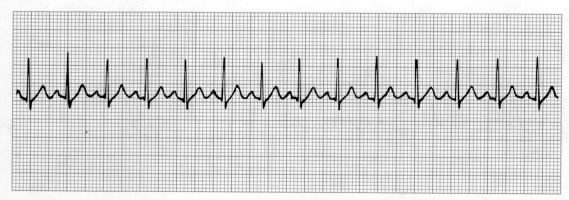

7. Rate _____   Rhythm _____

   P wave _____   PR interval _____

   QRS complex _____   Interpretation _____

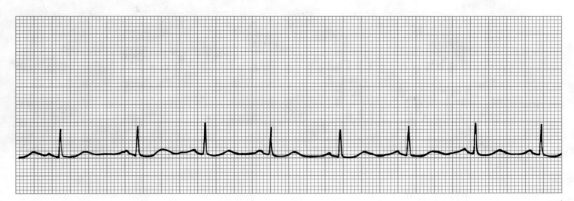

8. Rate _____   Rhythm _____
    P wave _____   PR interval _____
    QRS complex _____   Interpretation _____

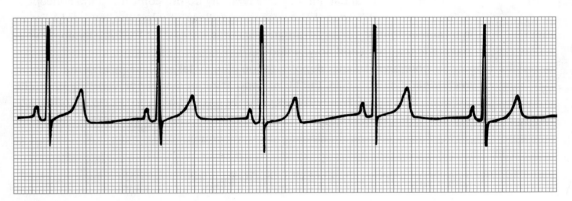

9. Rate _____   Rhythm _____
    P wave _____   PR interval _____
    QRS complex _____   Interpretation _____

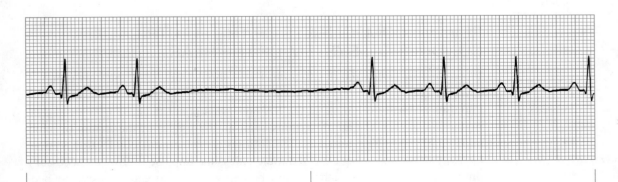

10. Rate _____   Rhythm _____
    P wave _____   PR interval _____
    QRS complex _____   Interpretation _____

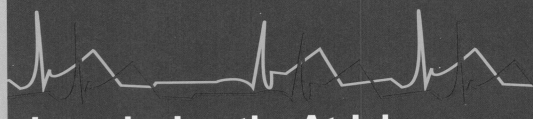

8

Objectives

Upon completion of this chapter, the student will be able to:

- Explain the origin of the atrial rhythms
- Recall the components of the electrical conduction system of the heart
- Identify a wandering atrial pacemaker rhythm, including EKG characteristics
- Describe a premature atrial contraction rhythm, including EKG characteristics
- Identify an atrial flutter rhythm, including EKG characteristics
- Recognize an atrial fibrillation rhythm, including EKG characteristics
- Describe supraventricular tachycardia, including EKG characteristics
- Recognize EKG characteristics of Wolff-Parkinson-White syndrome
- Discuss the clinical significance of the atrial rhythms

Introducing the Atrial Rhythms

INTRODUCTION

In our discussion of the sinus rhythms in Chapter 7, we examined rhythms originating in the normal place, the SA node. Beginning with this chapter, we will investigate rhythms that originate outside the SA node—away from the heart's primary pacemaker.

Remember that a reaction to, or tolerance of, a particular dysrhythmia is specific to the individual patient. Patients typically do not conform to the concept of a "one size fits all" adage! Therefore, regardless of what the textbooks list as typical reactions to certain dysrhythmias, it is imperative that you evaluate your patient in the "here and now" mind-set.

Although ventricular depolarization usually takes place in a normal fashion with atrial dysrhythmias, the atrial depolarization sequence depends upon the atrial rhythm. Atrial dysrhythmias occur as a result of hypoxia, myocardial ischemia, chronic congestive heart failure, valvular disease, or some combination of these.

ORIGIN OF THE ATRIAL RHYTHMS

If the SA node fails to generate an impulse, the atrial tissues or areas in the internodal pathways may initiate an impulse. When this occurs, the group of dysrhythmias produced is referred to as **atrial dysrhythmias**. Although atrial dysrhythmias are generally not considered life-threatening or lethal, careful and deliberate assessment of the patient must be a continuous process, as with all dysrhythmias.

REVIEW: COMPONENTS OF THE ELECTRICAL CONDUCTION SYSTEM OF THE HEART

When dealing with atrial dysrhythmias, you should remember that this group of rhythms does not directly pertain to the SA node. Although you learned that impulses normally originate in the SA node, this is not the case with atrial dysrhythmias. Rather, the atrial rhythms begin in the tissues of the atrium or internodal pathways. The impulse then follows the electrical conduction system pathway in the normal or expected route unless the impulse follows an **accessory pathway**. An accessory pathway may be defined as an irregular muscle connection between the atria and ventricles that bypasses the atrioventricular (AV) node. Traveling from the atria to the AV node, the impulse continues through the bundle of His, the left and right bundle branches, and the Purkinje network and terminates in the ventricular muscle wall.

atrial dysrhythmias the group of dysrhythmias produced when the SA node fails to generate an impulse and the atrial tissues or areas in the internodal pathways initiate an impulse

accessory pathway irregular muscle connection between the atria and ventricles that bypasses the AV node

3/24/16

WANDERING ATRIAL PACEMAKER RHYTHM

Wandering atrial pacemaker rhythms, also called wandering pacemaker or **WAP**, occur when pacemaker sites wander, or travel, from the SA node to other pacemaker sites in the atria, the internodal pathways, or the AV node. The SA node remains the basic pacemaker in the wandering pacemaker rhythms. For a diagnosis of wandering atrial pacemaker, observation of at least three different P waves on an EKG strip or cardiac monitor is required.

Wandering atrial pacemaker rhythms may be considered variants of sinus dysrhythmia rhythms. The size and shape of the P waves varies according to the site of origin, and there is a notable change in morphology from beat to beat. P waves may appear as upright, inverted, or absent waveforms. The absence of P waves in this rhythm may indicate that the P wave is buried in the QRS complex.

The PR interval (PRI) may be regular, but will sometimes vary on the basis of the point of origin. Causes of WAP vary: The rhythm may be a normal phenomenon (particularly in the aged or the very young) or the rhythm may be linked to underlying heart disease. At times, the rhythm may be simply a manifestation of the vagal effects of respirations. As with other rhythms, WAP may be a result of drug toxicity, especially with digitalis therapy.

Generally, a WAP rhythm produces no symptoms and can be recognized only by EKG observation. Although this rhythm is usually benign, it is wise to remember that it may indicate myocardial irritability and may thus require treatment. The potential for this rhythm to progress to more serious dysrhythmias cannot be ignored.

A variant of the WAP rhythm is **multifocal atrial tachycardia (MAT)**. When the rate of the WAP rhythm reaches 100 BPM or greater, the rhythm is called multifocal atrial tachycardia, or MAT. Although the MAT rhythm may be confused with atrial fibrillation, you should note that P waves will usually be visible in the MAT rhythm. Most often, MAT is observed in patients with advanced chronic obstructive pulmonary disease, digoxin toxicity, and electrolyte imbalances. Treatment of the underlying disorder may result in cessation of the MAT rhythm.

Now that we've discussed the notable features of a wandering atrial pacemaker rhythm, let's go back to the five-step approach to interpreting this rhythm. We'll ask the five questions that will enable us to identify the rhythm definitively and correctly. (See ■ **Table 8–1** and ■ **Figures 8–1a** and **b**.)

In reference to Figure 8–1a, you should note the heart rate as 50 BPM, the rhythm is regular, P wave is present, upright, and variable, the PRIs are variable depending on the site shifts, and the QRS is 0.08 seconds. These findings should validate a Wandering Atrial Pacemaker.

wandering atrial pacemaker (WAP) rhythms occur when pacemaker sites wander, or travel, from the SA node to other pacemaker sites in the atria, the internodal pathways, or the AV node

multifocal atrial tachycardia (MAT) rhythm created when the rate of the wandering atrial pacemaker rhythm reaches 100 BPM or greater

TABLE 8–1 Wandering atrial pacemaker rhythm

Questions 1–5	Answers
1. What is the rate?	Usually 60–100 BPM
2. What is the rhythm?	May be slightly irregular
3. Is there a P wave before each QRS? Are the P waves upright and uniform?	Change in shape, size, and location from beat to beat
4. What is the length of the PR interval?	Variable, depending on site shifts
5. Do all the QRS complexes look alike? What is the length of the QRS complexes?	Yes Usually less than 0.12 sec (3 small squares)

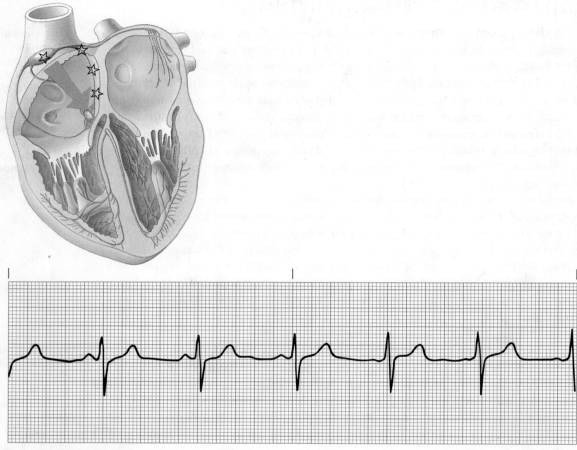

FIGURE 8–1a. Wandering atrial pacemaker rhythm

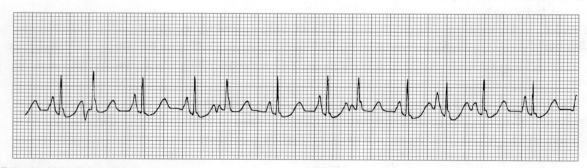

FIGURE 8–1b. Multifocal atrial tachycardia

In reference to Figure 8–1b, you should note the heart rate as 120 BPM, the rhythm is irregular, P wave is present, upright and variable, the PRI is variable, and the QRS is 0.04 seconds. These findings should validate Multifocal Atrial Tachycardia.

Recall that changes in the appearance of the P waves is the hallmark indicator in the diagnosis of WAP rhythms. **Remember . . . always monitor your patient's clinical condition!!**

3/25/16

PREMATURE ATRIAL CONTRACTIONS (COMPLEXES)

A single, electrical impulse that originates outside the SA node in the atria is called a **premature atrial contraction (PAC)**. This individual complex arises earlier than the next expected complex of the underlying rhythm, or prematurely. Quite often, a PAC will occur in an underlying sinus rhythm that may appear regular and within normal limits except for the presence of the PAC.

*We should note here that, although the word contraction is commonly used to describe this premature beat, all EKG strips and complexes represent only the **electrical** activity in the heart—not the **mechanical** activity. For this reason, it may be more appropriate to learn the term premature atrial complex rather than premature atrial contraction.*

Premature complexes can occur in the atria, the AV junction, or the ventricles. Simply stated, a premature beat is a complex that arises earlier than the next expected beat. In the process of analyzing an EKG strip, one may note that an extra complex is present or out of place. The next step then, is to decide on the site of origin of the extra complex. Normally, we expect the QRS of a PAC to be of normal size, shape, and duration.

An incomplete, or noncompensatory, pause often follows a PAC. This occurs because a PAC will usually cause the SA node to depolarize prematurely and will thus reset the SA node. The underlying rhythm, or cadence, of the heart is interrupted because of the premature atrial beat. After the noncompensatory pause, the underlying rhythm of the heart returns and continues until the next PAC occurs. Note the noncompensatory pause in ■ **Figure 8–2**.

premature atrial contraction (PAC) a single, electrical impulse that originates outside the SA node in the atria

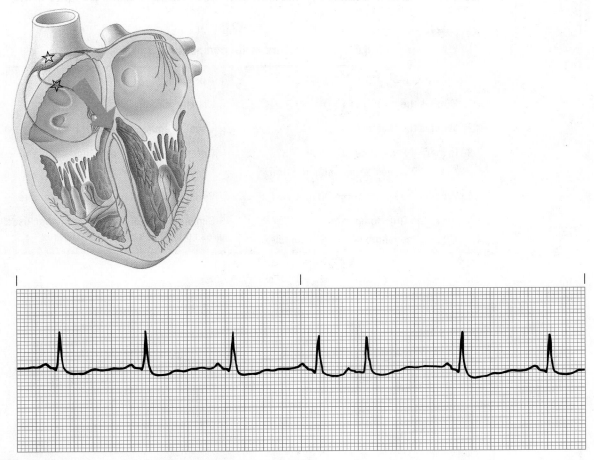

FIGURE 8–2. Premature atrial complex with noncompensatory pause

During your initial education in interpreting EKGs, it may be wise to remember that the PACs look very much like the normal complexes of the underlying rhythm. In Chapter 10, we will learn that this is not true of premature ventricular complexes. PACs may occur in any rhythm, but they are much easier to identify in any bradycardic rhythm.

PACs sometimes occur in patterns, such as pairs (two sequential PACs), atrial bigeminy (every other beat is a PAC), or atrial trigeminy (every third beat is a PAC). When you are counting the rate of a rhythm containing a PAC, it is important to remember that you should note the entire count of R waves of the PAC.

PACs may be caused by many different events. Causes of PACs may include the use of stimulants (caffeine, alcohol), hypoxia, increased sympathetic tone, imbalances of electrolytes, digitalis toxicity, or underlying cardiovascular disease. In some cases, isolated PACs may occur without cause.

Because this discussion is our first mention of *premature* beats or complexes, this is an appropriate time for you to recognize a very important fact—when any premature beat occurs more than six times per minute (min), the dysrhythmia assumes more importance and is called *frequent*. For instance, the rhythm may be called sinus bradycardia with frequent PACs. An increase in the frequency of premature beats indicates significant irritability of myocardial tissues and becomes a definite cause for concern. Be aware that more serious dysrhythmias may develop in the presence of frequent premature beats.

Now that we've examined the prominent characteristics of a PAC, let's explore the five-step approach to interpreting this rhythm. We'll ask the five questions that will enable us to identify the rhythm definitively and correctly. (See ■ **Table 8–2** and ■ **Figure 8–3**.)

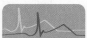 **TABLE 8–2 Premature atrial complexes**

Questions 1–5	Answers
1. What is the rate?	Usually normal
2. What is the rhythm?	Usually regular, except for PAC
3. Is there a P wave before each QRS? Are the P waves upright and uniform?	Differs in shape, size, and location from normal P waves of rhythm
4. What is the length of the PR interval?	Variable, depending on pacemaker site
5. Do all the QRS complexes look alike? What is the length of the QRS complexes?	Similar to QRS of underlying rhythm; usually less than 0.12 sec (3 small squares)

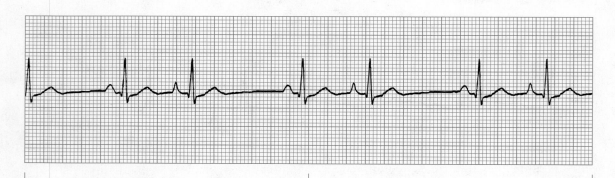

FIGURE 8–3. Premature atrial complexes

In reference to Figure 8–3, you should note the heart rate as 70 BPM, the rhythm is irregular, P wave is present and upright, the PRI is 0.16 seconds, and the QRS is 0.06 seconds. These findings should validate Premature Atrial Complexes.

Remember that the PAC often appears as an "ectopic" (or out-of-place) beat in an otherwise regular rhythm. **Remember . . . always monitor your patient's clinical condition!**

REENTRY DYSRHYTHMIAS

Reentry can be defined as the reactivation of myocardial tissue for a second or subsequent time by the same electrical impulse. Although reentry is a common dysrhythmic mechanism, it is a complicated event. This concept can be thought of as a "short circuit" of the heart's electrical conduction system.

Reentry develops when the course of an electrical impulse is delayed or blocked in one or more segments of the heart's electrical conduction system. Because of this delay, the electrical impulse is allowed to travel in only one direction (unilateral). As the impulse moves in a cycle throughout the heart tissue, a series of fast depolarization ensues. (See ■ **Figure 8–4**.)

Causes of reentry due to conduction delays or blocks include hyperkalemia, myocardial ischemia, and certain antidysrhythmic medications. Specific rhythms associated with reentry include atrial flutter, atrial fibrillation, paroxysmal supraventricular tachycardia, and premature atrial complexes.

reentry reactivation of myocardial tissue for a second or subsequent time by the same electrical impulse

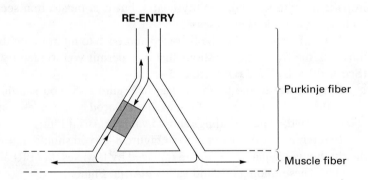

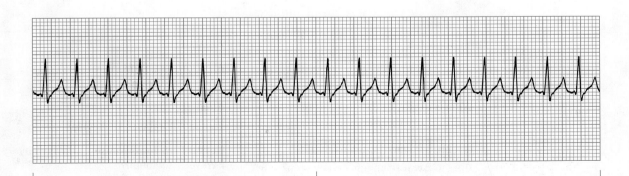

FIGURE 8–4. Reentry is a phenomenon usually created by a one-way block that causes a wave of depolarization to be rapidly propagated in a circular motion. Upper: Schematic drawing. Lower: EKG tracing.

ATRIAL FLUTTER RHYTHM

Another common atrial dysrhythmia is called atrial flutter. Atrial flutter is characterized by the presence of regular atrial activity with a picket-fence or sawtooth pattern. Think *sawtooth!* This rhythm is often a favorite of students who are initially learning EKG interpretation because it is generally easy to recognize.

When a single irritable site in the atria initiates many electrical impulses at a rapid rate, the rhythm is called **atrial flutter**. Normal P waves are not produced in atrial flutter because electrical impulses are conducted throughout the atria at a very rapid rate. Rather than the presence of normally appearing P waves, flutter (or sawtooth) waves, also known as F waves, are patterned.

The AV node plays a very important role in atrial flutter rhythms: It truly becomes the "gatekeeper" to the ventricles. The ventricular response rate is based on the number of impulses that the AV node accepts. In other words, if every other flutter impulse is blocked by the AV node, the conduction ratio becomes 2 to 1—there will be two atrial contractions for each ventricular contraction. If the AV node conducts only one of every four atrial contractions, the conduction ratio is 4 to 1; thus an atrial rate of 300 BPM will parallel a ventricular rate of 75 BPM. If the conduction ratio changes or varies frequently, an irregular ventricular rate will result. In addition, if the conduction ratio is 2 to 1, the F waves may be more difficult to recognize. Atrial flutter with a ventricular rate of less than 60 BPM is atrial flutter with a **slow ventricular response**. A ventricular rate of 100 to 150 BPM is atrial flutter with a **rapid ventricular response**.

Causes of atrial flutter include acute myocardial infarction, hypoxia, digitalis toxicity, congestive heart failure, SA node disease, and pulmonary embolism. Atrial flutter may occur in patients with normal, healthy hearts, but it is most often seen in elderly patients with underlying chronic heart disease.

We will now examine the five-step approach to interpreting this rhythm. As always, you must ask the five basic questions that will permit you to identify this rhythm conclusively. (See ■ **Table 8–3** and ■ **Figure 8–5**.)

In reference to the topmost strip in Figure 8–5, you should note the heart rate as 80 BPM, the rhythm is regular, P waves are replaced by F waves, the PRI absent, and the QRS is 0.04 seconds. These findings should validate Atrial Flutter.

In reference to the lower strip in Figure 8–5, you should note the heart rate as 100 BPM, the rhythm is regular, P waves are replaced by F waves, the PRI absent, and the QRS is 0.04 seconds. These findings should validate Atrial Flutter.

atrial flutter when a single irritable site in the atria initiates many electrical impulses at a rapid rate, characterized by the presence of regular atrial activity with a picket-fence or sawtooth pattern

slow ventricular response a ventricular rate of less than 60 BPM

rapid ventricular response a ventricular rate of 100 to 150 BPM

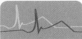

TABLE 8–3 Atrial flutter

Questions 1–5	Answers
1. What is the rate?	Atrial: 250–300 BPM Ventricular: variable
2. What is the rhythm?	Atrial: regular Ventricular: regular or irregular
3. Is there a P wave before each QRS? Are the P waves upright and uniform?	Normal P waves are absent; replaced by F waves (sawtooth)
4. What is the length of the PR interval?	Not measurable
5. Do all the QRS complexes look alike? What is the Length of the QRS Complexes?	Usually less than 0.12 sec (3 small squares)

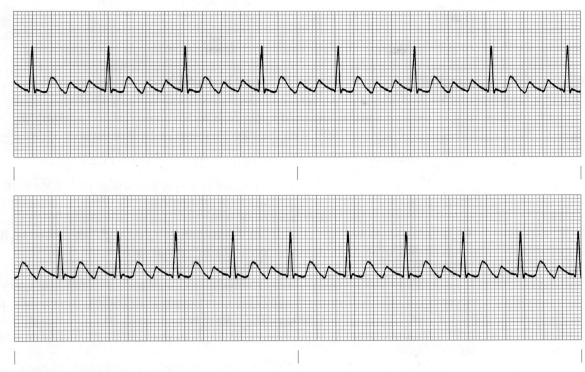

FIGURE 8–5. Atrial flutter

Recall that the **key** to interpreting atrial flutter is the presence of a *sawtooth pattern*. **Remember . . . always monitor your patient's clinical condition!**

ATRIAL FIBRILLATION RHYTHM

Atrial fibrillation is one of the most common atrial dysrhythmias encountered in elderly patients. Typically, atrial fibrillation presents with three definite characteristics. First, there is a notable absence of P waves in this rhythm. Second, P waves are replaced by *f* waves, or fibrillatory waves. Third, possibly the most obvious characteristic of atrial fibrillation is that the ventricular response rate is totally irregular—it is called an *irregular irregularity*. The QRS complexes in an atrial fibrillation rhythm are usually within normal limits.

When multiple disorganized ectopic atrial foci generate electrical activity at a very rapid rate (atrial rate varies from 350–750 BPM), **atrial fibrillation** results. The ventricular response rate is 140 to 200 BPM in the *untreated* atrial fibrillation rhythms. In this rhythm, multiple ectopic foci from within the atria are literally blitzing the AV node. It is pathophysiologically impossible for the AV node to handle or conduct each of these impulses. Consequently, the AV node allows impulses to enter the conduction system pathway completely at random. This random selection of impulse passage through the AV node accounts for the total irregularity of the rhythm called atrial fibrillation. In the truest sense of EKG interpretation, atrial fibrillation is an irregular irregularity in heart rhythm.

Frequently, we find ourselves shortening or abbreviating the pronunciation of this rhythm; however, I discourage my students from this practice because the abbreviated terms a-fib and v-fib sound very much alike but indicate *very different* rhythms. It's easier to be safe and take another millisecond to pronounce both words—atrial fibrillation!

As we address the causes of atrial fibrillation, it is important to note that this rhythm may be chronic in nature and is quite commonly associated with underlying heart diseases,

atrial fibrillation
when multiple disorganized ectopic atrial foci generate electrical activity at a very rapid rate (atrial rate varies from 350–750 BPM)

no insuficient blood flow to the heart muscle via coronary arteries.

non specific medical problem affecting joints 4 connective tissue

such as congestive heart failure or rheumatic heart disease. This rhythm may also be associated with acute myocardial infarction, common electrolyte imbalances, hypoxia, myocardial ischemia, or digitalis toxicity. It is important to note that atrial fibrillation also increases the risk of stroke thus many of the patients you encounter will be taking an anti-coagulant medication. *reduce blood clots.*

The goal of therapy when treating atrial fibrillation with a rapid ventricular response is to slow the ventricular response to somewhere within a range of 80 to 100 BPM. This can sometimes be accomplished with the careful, monitored administration of beta-blockers (example, Lopressor), calcium-channel blockers (example, Cardiazem), or cardiac glucosides (example, digoxin).

While considering this rhythm, one might visualize the atria as though they are "quivering." When this occurs, the atria do not contract productively. Thus the effectiveness of myocardial contraction is decreased because the atria are not forcefully filling the ventricles with blood. As with the majority of dysrhythmias, a new occurrence of atrial fibrillation is usually treated when discovered, as it can indicate an increase in irritability within the atrial tissue.

Recall now that irritability in myocardial tissue can signal progression to a more serious dysrhythmia. Ask yourself how well your patient is tolerating this rhythm. If your patient is clinically symptomatic and you elect to administer oxygen, do the symptoms abate after the oxygen is administered? If not, you must then consider what course of action to follow.

As we examine the five-step approach to interpreting this rhythm, contemplate your concerns about the clinical condition of an imagined patient and decisively identify this rhythm. Again, do not be shy or hesitant about asking for guidance if you falter during the initial trial of rhythm interpretation. Remember, there are no stupid questions. There are just questions that are unasked and thus unanswered. *Hint:* **Think "irregular irregularity"**—it just may be atrial fibrillation. (See ■ **Table 8–4** and ■ **Figure 8–6**.)

In reference to Figure 8–6, you should note the heart rate as 90 BPM, the rhythm is irregular, P waves are replaced by *f* waves, the PRI not discernible, and the QRS is 0.06 seconds. These findings should validate Atrial Fibrillation.

Recall that the **key** to interpreting atrial fibrillation is the **presence of an irregularly irregular pattern and an absence of P waves. Remember . . . always monitor your patient's clinical condition!**

TABLE 8–4 Atrial fibrillation

Questions 1–5	Answers
1. What is the rate?	Atrial: 350–400 BPM Ventricular: variable
2. What is the rhythm?	Irregularly irregular
3. Is there a P wave before each QRS? Are the P waves upright and uniform?	Normal P waves are absent; replaced by f waves
4. What is the length of the PR interval?	Not discernible
5. Do all the QRS complexes look alike? What is the length of the QRS complexes?	Yes Usually less than 0.10 sec

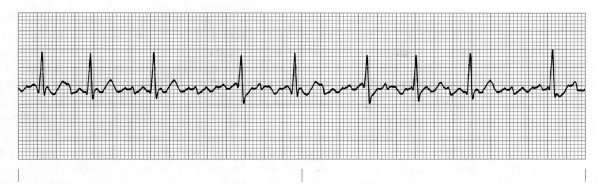

FIGURE 8–6. Atrial fibrillation

SUPRAVENTRICULAR TACHYCARDIA RHYTHMS

Supraventricular tachycardia (SVT) is a general term that encompasses all fast (tachy-) dysrhythmias in which the heart rate is greater than 100 BPM. Technically, even sinus tachycardia is a supraventricular tachycardia, in that it is a rhythm arising above (supra) the ventricles (ventricular). Generally, we think of SVT as the "big umbrella" title of dysrhythmias, under which cascades a host of specific rhythms: paroxysmal supraventricular tachycardia (PSVT), paroxysmal atrial tachycardia (PAT), atrial tachycardia (AT), paroxysmal junctional tachycardia (PJT), multifocal atrial tachycardia (MAT), and junctional tachycardia (JT). Thus, the term supraventricular tachycardia technically applies to any tachycardia rhythm originating above the ventricle.

It is wise to attempt to identify where the rhythm is originating in order to get a good idea of which type of SVT you are observing. Differential diagnosis of the exact type of SVT being observed is not critical in the emergent situation and should never delay patient care. Look at your patient. **Treat the patient, not the monitor!**

The term **paroxysmal** refers to a sudden onset or cessation or both. In order to label a rhythm correctly as paroxysmal, it is critical that the sudden onset or cessation be observed on the cardiac monitor. Only then, in the strictest sense, can the rhythm be **correctly** identified as paroxysmal in nature. Typically, bouts of PSVT begin and end abruptly. Notably, these bouts may continue for several hours or for only a few seconds.

Supraventricular tachycardia occurs when a rapid atrial ectopic focus overrides the SA node and become the heart's primary pacemaker. Supraventricular tachycardia can resemble a rapid sinus tachycardia; thus careful calculation of the heart rate is important. Recall that sinus tachycardia seldom exceeds 160 to 170 BPM at the high-rate range. In both these dysrhythmias, the QRS complexes are typically normal in appearance. When P waves are present, they have a consistent relationship with the QRS complexes. In SVT rhythms, P waves are often hidden in the T waves of the preceding complex and thus may be difficult, if not impossible, to discern.

Causes of the SVT rhythms are similar, in part, to the causes of other atrial dysrhythmias. Although SVT is not a common finding in the setting of an acute myocardial infarction, this rhythm may be associated with underlying cardiovascular diseases such as rheumatic heart disease and atherosclerotic cardiovascular disease. Supraventricular tachycardia may occur in a healthy person and can result from overexertion, stress, hypoxia, excessive use of stimulants, or hypokalemia.

Methods utilized to stimulate baroreceptors (located in the internal carotid and aortic arch) are called **vagal maneuvers**. When these receptors are stimulated, the vagus nerve releases acetylcholine, resulting in slowing of the heart rate. Examples of vagal maneuvers

supraventricular tachycardia (SVT) general term that encompasses all fast (tachy-) dysrhythmias in which the heart rate is greater than 100 BPM

paroxysmal refers to a sudden onset or cessation or both

vagal maneuvers methods utilized to stimulate baroreceptors (located in the internal carotid and aortic arch); when these receptors are stimulated, the vagus nerve releases acetylcholine, resulting in slowing of the heart rate

include asking the patient to bear down (as in an attempt to move the bowels), cough, or squat and using carotid sinus massage. (Carotid sinus massage must be avoided with older patients and only performed unilaterally.)

Let's examine the five-step approach to interpreting this rhythm. *Hint:* **Think: What is the heart rate, and can I see definite P waves?** (See ■ **Table 8–5** and ■ **Figure 8–7.**)

In reference to the topmost strip in Figure 8–7, you should note the heart rate as 250 BPM, the rhythm is regular, P waves are not discernible, the PRI absent, and the QRS is 0.04 seconds. These findings should validate Supraventricular Tachycardia.

In reference to the lower strip in Figure 8–7, you should note the heart rate as 170, the rhythm is regular, P waves are not discernible, the PRI absent, and the QRS is 0.04 seconds. These findings should validate Supraventricular Tachycardia.

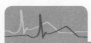 **TABLE 8–5 Supraventricular tachycardia**

Questions 1–5	Answers
1. What is the rate?	Atrial: 150–250 BPM
	Ventricular: 150–250 BPM
2. What is the rhythm?	Regular
3. Is there a P wave before each QRS? Are the P waves upright and uniform?	Usually not discernible, especially at the high-rate range
4. What is the length of the PR interval?	Usually not discernible
5. Do all the QRS complexes look alike? What is the Length of the QRS Complexes?	Yes Usually less than 0.10 sec

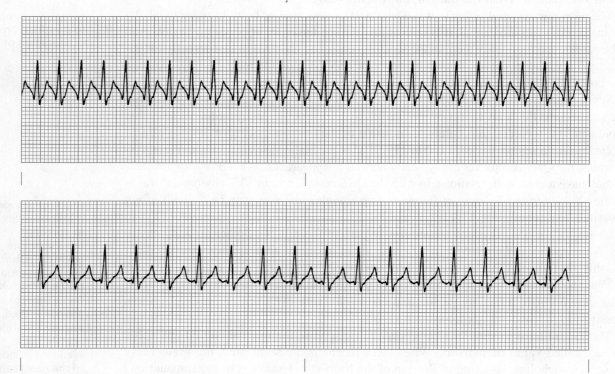

FIGURE 8–7. Supraventricular tachycardia

Remember that the patient who is experiencing PSVT may complain of a feeling that his or her heart is running away or racing. **Remember: It is critical to determine whether the patient is symptomatic or nonsymptomatic; therefore, always monitor your patient's clinical condition!**

WOLFF-PARKINSON-WHITE SYNDROME

In the 1930s, an American physician, Louis Wolff; an English cardiologist, Sir John Parkinson; and an American cardiologist, Paul Dudley White, identified the preexcitation syndrome called **Wolff-Parkinson-White (WPW) syndrome**. This atrioventricular conduction disorder is characterized by two AV conduction pathways and is often identified by a characteristic delta wave seen on an electrocardiogram at the beginning of the QRS complex. In most patients, WPW is not related to other heart abnormalities. WPW can occur at any age, is often first noted in childhood, but may not be diagnosed until adulthood in some patients. Symptoms of WPW are often abrupt and may include chest discomfort, palpitations, and occasionally fainting.

abnormal heart beat

In WPW syndrome, the QRS complex is greater than 0.10 seconds because the ventricles are stimulated by an impulse that originated outside the normal conduction pathway. Wolff-Parkinson-White syndrome is thought to be congenital. If P waves are identifiable in WPW rhythms, the PR interval may be 0.12 seconds or longer because the AV node is bypassed. This disorder is associated with a high incidence of tachydysrhythmias. Treatment of WPW, if required, is based on the underlying rhythm as well as the patient's clinical condition. (See ■ **Figure 8–8**.)

> **Wolff-Parkinson-White (WPW) syndrome** preexcitation syndrome and atrioventricular conduction disorder characterized by two AV conduction pathways and is often identified by a characteristic delta wave seen on an electrocardiogram at the beginning of the QRS complex

CLINICAL SIGNIFICANCE OF ATRIAL RHYTHMS

3/24/16

Wandering atrial pacemaker rhythm

Wandering atrial pacemaker rhythms are not typically clinically significant. The patient is usually asymptomatic, but it should be noted that WAP can be a precursor of other atrial dysrhythmias. This rhythm may be caused by digitalis toxicity; therefore, the patient's digitalis blood level must be closely monitored, and the medication should be adjusted accordingly.

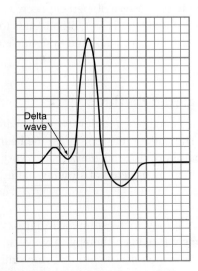

Delta wave

FIGURE 8–8. Delta wave of Wolff-Parkinson-White syndrome

Premature atrial contraction (complex)

In a person with a healthy heart, isolated PACs are not significant. As with many other dysrhythmias, PACs may be corrected by identifying and treating the underlying cause.

Frequent PACs (more than 6 per min) may signify underlying heart disease and may initiate other atrial dysrhythmias, such as atrial fibrillation, atrial tachycardia, PSVT, or atrial flutter.

Atrial flutter rhythm

The clinical significance of atrial flutter is directly related to the patient's clinical condition. If the ventricular rate is normal, the rhythm is generally well tolerated. If the ventricular response rate is fast, a decrease in cardiac output may occur, resulting in symptoms. As ventricular response rates increase, the patient may complain of dizziness, weakness, chest pain, or palpitations. Because atrial flutter causes ineffective contractions of the atria, the patient may develop pooling of the blood in the atria, causing susceptibility to the formation of thrombus. In cases of rapid ventricular response rates, treatment may be directed toward decreasing the ventricular rate with medication. If the patient's symptoms progress and the patient becomes hemodynamically unstable, cardioversion may be indicated.

The initial setting for synchronized cardioversion is 50 to 100 joules (J) in atrial flutter rhythms. Recall also that oxygen therapy is the first and most important therapy for patients who are exhibiting signs or symptoms of compromised cardiac output, regardless of the cause.

Atrial fibrillation rhythm

If the patient does not exhibit signs or symptoms, no treatment may be required. This is often the case in patients with controlled atrial fibrillation. Cardiac output can fall, due to ventricular response rates of less than 60 BPM. In cases of rapid ventricular response rates, treatment may be directed toward decreasing the ventricular rate with the administration of medications. If the patient's symptoms progress and the patient becomes hemodynamically unstable, cardioversion may be indicated and should be initiated at 120 to 200 J, depending on the physician's preference.

It is wise to keep in mind that the atria do not empty sufficiently in rapid atrial fibrillation rhythms. Lack of atrial activity causes a 30 percent decrease in cardiac output. Because the **atrial kick** (the final phase of diastole) is lost, blood tends to stagnate in the atria. These patients are at risk for the development of atrial and systemic emboli and must be carefully monitored.

atrial kick the final phase of diastole, atrial contraction forces remaining blood into the ventricles: provides 15 percent to 30 percent of ventricular filling

Supraventricular tachycardia rhythms

Supraventricular rhythms may occur in a patient with a healthy heart and may be well tolerated for short intervals. The patient may complain the heart is racing or running away (a common description of palpitations) and may appear very anxious or excited. If the patient is symptomatic, treatment is directed at slowing the heart rate by the use of vagal maneuvers, drug therapy, such as adenosine, or synchronized cardioversion (initial setting of 100 J).

Prolonged episodes of SVT may increase myocardial oxygen demand and may thus increase the need for supplemental oxygen therapy. Always administer oxygen to patients who are exhibiting any signs or symptoms of cardiac compromise. To determine the appropriate course of treatment, you must observe and assess your patient's clinical condition.

CHAPTER 8

 SUMMARY

Dysrhythmias that originate in the atrial tissues, or in the internodal pathways, are referred to as atrial dysrhythmias. Atrial dysrhythmias arise from many causes, including hypoxia, ischemia, and atrial enlargement secondary to congestive heart failure. As with the treatment and management of all patients exhibiting dysrhythmias, excellent patient assessment skills are critically important.

 KEY POINTS TO REMEMBER

1. Atrial dysrhythmias occur when the SA node fails to generate impulses; other areas within the atria take over as pacemaker sites.

2. Atrial dysrhythmias are generally not considered to be life-threatening events.

3. Wandering atrial pacemaker rhythms may occur when the pacemaker site wanders, or "travels," through the atria.

4. The WAP rhythm strip must illustrate three different P wave configurations in order to be definitively identified as *wandering*.

5. A variant of wandering atrial pacemaker rhythm is called multifocal atrial tachycardia (MAT).

6. Remember: It is critical that you always determine whether the patient is symptomatic or nonsymptomatic; that is, monitor your patient's clinical condition.

7. Premature complexes, such as a premature atrial contraction, can occur in the atria, AV junction or the ventricles.

8. EKG strips represent only the electrical activity in the heart and not the mechanical activity.

9. Atrial flutter occurs when a single irritable site in the atria initiates many electrical impulses at a rapid rate; as a result, flutter, or sawtooth, waves are formed.

10. Atrial fibrillation is one of the most common atrial dysrhythmias encountered in the elderly and occurs when multiple disorganized ectopic atrial foci generate electrical activity at a rapid rate.

11. A generalized term that encompasses all fast or tachydysrhythmias when the heart rate is greater than 100 BPM is supraventricular tachycardia (SVT).

12. A rhythm that refers to sudden onset or cessation is paroxysmal.

13. Vagal maneuvers refer to methods utilized to stimulate the vagus nerve resulting in slowing of the heart rate.

14. Prolonged episodes of SVT may increase myocardial oxygen demands.

 REVIEW QUESTIONS

1. Vagal maneuvers are performed to:
   a. Slow the heart rate
   b. Dilate the coronary arteries
   c. Reduce ventricular irritability
   d. Improve conduction through the AV node

2. The coronary arteries receive oxygenated blood from the:
   a. Aorta
   b. Coronary sinus
   c. Pulmonary veins
   d. Pulmonary arteries

3. When any premature beat occurs more than six times per minute, the dysrhythmia assumes more importance and is called:
   a. Regular
   b. Frequent
   c. Irregular
   d. Continual

4. The initial setting for cardioversion is _____ J in atrial flutter rhythms.
   a. 200–250
   b. 150–200
   c. 200–300
   d. 50–100

5. The electrocardiogram is used to:
   a. Determine pulse rate
   b. Detect valvular dysfunction
   c. Evaluate electrical activity in the heart
   d. Determine whether the heart is beating

6. Most atrial fibrillation waves are not followed by a QRS complex because the:
   a. Impulses are initiated in the left ventricle
   b. Stimuli are not strong enough to be conducted
   c. Ventricle can receive only 120 stimuli in 1 min
   d. AV junction is unable to conduct all the excitation impulses

7. Supraventricular rhythm means that the impulse, or stimulus, arises above the ventricles.
   a. True
   b. False

8. PAT is a sudden onset of atrial tachycardia.
   a. True
   b. False

9. The T wave on the EKG strip represents:
   a. Rest period
   b. Bundle of His
   c. Atrial contraction
   d. Ventricular contraction

10. When interpreting dysrhythmias, you must remember that the most important key is the:
    a. PR interval
    b. Rate and rhythm
    c. Presence of dysrhythmias
    d. Patient's clinical appearance

11. Premature atrial complexes may occur in any rhythm but are much easier to identify in any bradycardic rhythm.
    a. True
    b. False

12. For a diagnosis of wandering atrial pacemaker, observation of at least _____ different P waves is required.
    a. Two
    b. Three
    c. Four
    d. Six

13. Methods used to stimulate baroreceptors (located in the internal carotid and aortic arch) are called _____ maneuvers.
    a. Reflex
    b. Vasal
    c. Vagal
    d. Sinus

14. When a single irritable site in the atria initiates many electrical impulses at a rapid rate, the rhythm is called:
    a. Sinus rhythm
    b. Atrial flutter
    c. Atrial fibrillation
    d. Atrial tachycardia

15. SVT may occur in a healthy person and can result from:
    a. Overexertion
    b. Hypoxia
    c. Hypokalemia
    d. All the above

REVIEW STRIPS

1. Rate _____   Rhythm _____

   P wave _____   PR interval _____

   QRS complex _____   Interpretation _____

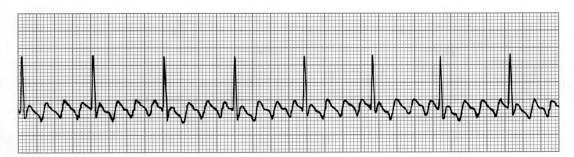

2. Rate _____   Rhythm _____

    P wave _____   PR interval _____

    QRS complex _____   Interpretation _____

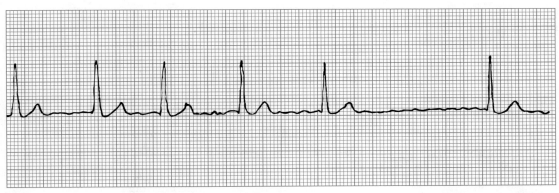

3. Rate _____   Rhythm _____

    P wave _____   PR interval _____

    QRS complex _____   Interpretation _____

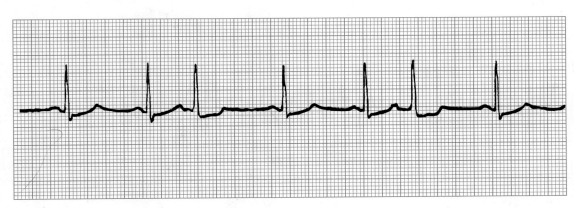

4. Rate _____   Rhythm _____

    P wave _____   PR interval _____

    QRS complex _____   Interpretation _____

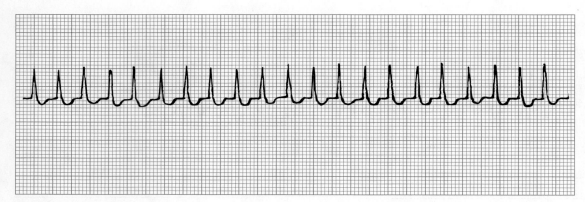

5. Rate _____   Rhythm _____

   P wave _____   PR interval _____

   QRS complex _____   Interpretation _____

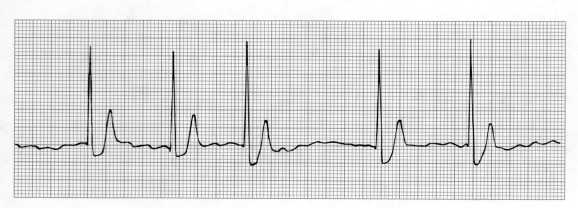

6. Rate _____   Rhythm _____

   P wave _____   PR interval _____

   QRS complex _____   Interpretation _____

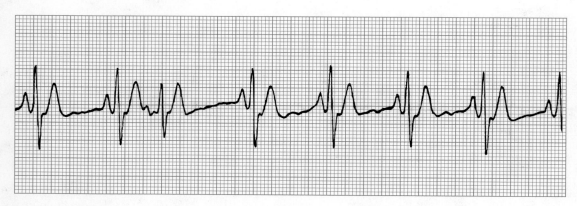

7. Rate _____   Rhythm _____

   P wave _____   PR interval _____

   QRS complex _____   Interpretation _____

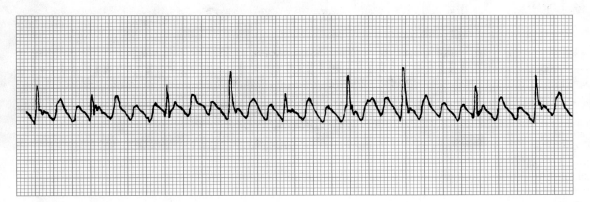

8. Rate _____   Rhythm _____

   P wave _____   PR interval _____

   QRS complex _____   Interpretation _____

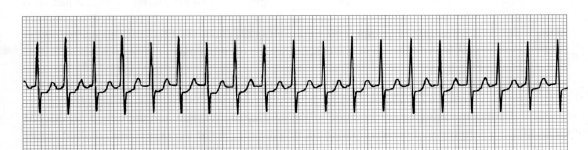

9. Rate _____   Rhythm _____

   P wave _____   PR interval _____

   QRS complex _____   Interpretation _____

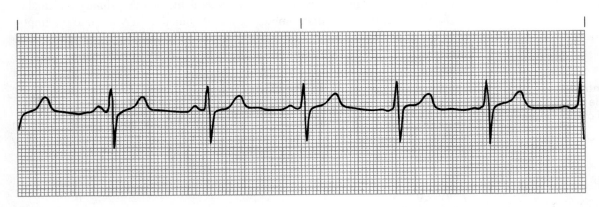

10. Rate _____   Rhythm _____

    P wave _____   PR interval _____

    QRS complex _____   Interpretation _____

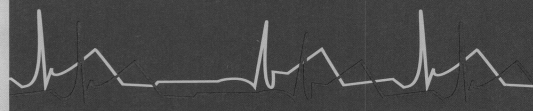

9

Objectives

Upon completion of this chapter, the student will be able to:

- Discuss the origin of junctional rhythms
- Recall the components of the electrical conduction system
- Identify premature junctional contractions, including EKG characteristics
- Recognize a junctional escape rhythm, including EKG characteristics
- Identify an accelerated junctional rhythm, including EKG characteristics
- Explain a junctional tachycardia rhythm, including EKG characteristics
- Discuss the clinical significance of the junctional rhythms

junctional rhythms rhythms that are initiated in the area of the AV junction

retrograde contrary (or opposite) to the normal expected path of movement

Introducing the Junctional Rhythms

INTRODUCTION

In Chapters 7 and 8, we discussed sinus rhythms and atrial rhythms. We learned that the sinoatrial (SA) node is the primary pacemaker in the heart and that impulses sometimes arise from the atria. For various reasons, such as drug toxicity or underlying cardiac disease, the SA node and the atria may fail to initiate electrical impulses. If this failure develops, the secondary pacemaker of the heart, the atrioventricular (AV) junction, will assume the role of pacing the heart.

It may be helpful for you to recognize that all junctional dysrhythmias contain several similar EKG features. These common features include P waves that are inverted or absent, a PR interval that is usually less than 0.12 seconds in duration, and QRS complexes that are within normal limits.

ORIGIN OF JUNCTIONAL RHYTHMS

Rhythms that are initiated in the area of the AV junction are called **junctional rhythms**. Formerly, rhythms originating in the AV node were called nodal rhythms. Technically, and in reference to pathophysiology of the heart, junctional is a more accurate term than nodal. Thus, in this chapter, we discuss the more common junctional rhythms. Although junctional rhythms are not considered lethal or life-threatening rhythms, you should recall that *patient assessment* is the most important indicator of the clinical significance of any dysrhythmia.

REVIEW OF THE ELECTRICAL CONDUCTION SYSTEM

We learned earlier in this text that the SA node is the heart's primary pacemaker. If the SA node fails to initiate impulses, the AV junction may assume the important role of pacing the heart. In the case of a junctional rhythm, the atria will actually still contract before the ventricles. When the AV junction becomes the dominant pacemaker of the heart, the atria may or may not be stimulated. In order for the atria to be activated, the electrical impulses must travel in a **retrograde** conduction (backward) direction from the AV junction. In retrograde conduction, the conduction comes from the ventricles or from the AV node into and through the atria. Therefore, the presence, absence, and location of P waves become key factors in the interpretation of junctional rhythms.

P WAVES

Recall now that we normally expect to see P waves *before* each QRS complex. However, because the electrical impulse in a junctional rhythm is traveling away from the positive electrode in Leads II and III, the P wave will be inverted or negative. At times, the P wave will not be seen, if atrial depolarization and ventricular depolarization occur simultaneously. In this case, the P wave is hidden in the QRS complex. At other times, the atria will depolarize after the ventricles have depolarized. When this occurs, an inverted P wave will appear *after* the QRS complex.

On the basis of this information, you should remember that a P wave may be seen before or after the QRS complex, or it may not be visible at all, in a junctional rhythm. The impulse produces a narrow QRS complex because the ventricle is depolarized using the normal conduction pathway. You should recognize that the retrograde movement of the electrical impulses in junctional dysrhythmias accounts for all three of the distinctive changes in the P waves.

PREMATURE JUNCTIONAL CONTRACTIONS

Formerly called premature nodal contractions (PNCs), **premature junctional contractions (PJCs)** are initiated from a single site in the AV junction or bundle of His/Purkinje system and arise earlier than the next anticipated complex of the underlying rhythm. If the SA node is depolarized by the ectopic beat, a noncompensatory pause occurs. Recall now that a **noncompensatory pause** (as we learned in our discussion of PACs in Chapter 8) is the pause that occurs after an ectopic beat, when the SA node is depolarized. Because of this noncompensatory pause, the underlying rhythm of the heart is interrupted. Premature junctional contractions can also result in a **compensatory pause** (a pause that occurs after an ectopic beat in which the SA node is unaffected and the cadence of the heart is uninterrupted). Therefore, we recognize that PJCs can result in either a compensatory or a noncompensatory pause, depending on whether the SA node is influenced by the ectopic beat.

PJCs, or complexes, are less common than premature atrial complexes (PACs, discussed in Chapter 8) or premature ventricular contractions (PVCs, to be discussed in Chapter 10) and may occur in any rhythm. As with all ectopic beats, it is easier to identify PJCs when the rhythm is sinus or bradycardic. Also as with other premature beats, you should remember to determine the heart rate by counting the total number of R waves (including the R wave of the PJC). In addition, when interpreting a rhythm strip containing a PJC, you must determine the underlying rhythm. For example, a strip of sinus rhythm that includes one PJC is called *sinus rhythm with a PJC.*

Causes of PJCs may include fever, anxiety, exercise, drug effects, electrolyte imbalances, congestive heart failure (CHF), stimulants (such as caffeine and tobacco), hypoxia, or myocardial ischemia. PJCs may occur without any definite underlying cause. It is important to note that isolated occurrences of PJCs are not life-threatening. However, as with any dysrhythmia, the patient should be monitored closely because more serious dysrhythmias may be precipitated by ectopic foci.

Now, it's time to apply the five-step approach to rhythm analysis in order to recognize a PJC correctly. Remember: When analyzing a static (stationary, paper) strip, **always** study the strip from left to right. (See ■ **Table 9–1** and ■ **Figure 9–1.**)

In Figure 9–1, you should note the heart rate as 80 BPM, the rhythm is irregular, P wave is present and upright in normal complexes but absent in premature complexes, the PRI is 0.16 seconds in normal complexes and absent in premature complexes, and the QRS is 0.04 seconds. These findings should validate Sinus Rhythm with Premature Junctional Complexes.

Remember that the appearance of the P wave (inverted, absent, or occurring after the QRS) is the **key** to discerning the presence of premature junctional complexes. **Remember . . . always monitor your patient's clinical condition!**

premature junctional contractions (PJCs) initiate from a single site in the AV junction and arise earlier than the next anticipated complex of the underlying rhythm

noncompensatory pause the pause that occurs after an ectopic beat, when the SA node is depolarized

compensatory pause a pause that occurs after an ectopic beat in which the SA node is unaffected and the cadence of the heart is uninterrupted

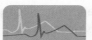

TABLE 9–1 Premature junctional complexes

Questions 1–5	Answers
1. What is the rate?	Rate of underlying rhythm, plus the PJC or PJCs
2. What is the rhythm?	Usually regular, except for premature beat (PJC)
3. Is there a P wave before each QRS?	Inverted or absent
Are the P waves upright and uniform?	May appear before or after the QRS
4. What is the length of the PR interval?	Usually less than 0.12 sec if P wave precedes QRS; absent if no P wave occurs before the QRS
5. Do all the QRS complexes look alike? What is the length of the QRS complexes?	Yes
	Less than 0.12 sec, if no defect in ventricular conduction

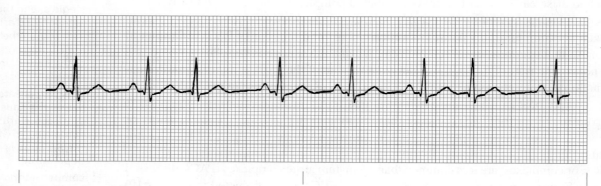

FIGURE 9–1. Premature junctional complexes

JUNCTIONAL ESCAPE RHYTHMS

If you recall our discussion of the electrical conduction system of the heart (Chapter 4), you will remember learning about the heart's pacemakers. We know that the heart is indeed an amazing organ. If, for any number of reasons, the SA node fails to generate an impulse or if the rate of impulse generation falls below that of the AV node, then the AV node/junction will assume the role of the pacemaker. When this occurs, the resulting rhythm is called a **junctional escape rhythm**. The ability of the AV node to assume this role is a safety feature of the heart. Recall now that the intrinsic rate of the AV node is 40 to 60 BPM.

If an isolated junctional beat occurs, it is called a *junctional escape beat (or complex)*. If a series of junctional escape beats occur, the rhythm is then called a *junctional escape rhythm*. This rhythm is also sometimes termed a junctional bradycardia when the rate falls below 40 BPM. Remember that, as we discussed earlier in this chapter, the P wave may not be seen if atrial and ventricular depolarization occur simultaneously.

Causes of junctional escape beats or junctional escape rhythm include SA node disease, hypoxia, increased parasympathetic (vagal) tone, certain cardiac drugs, and a complete heart block. A patient with a junctional escape rhythm may be symptomatic or asymptomatic. If the patient is symptomatic, the treatment will be based on the underlying cause of the dysrhythmia.

The five-step approach should now be applied to the rhythm represented in ■ **Table 9–2** and ■ **Figure 9–2**.

junctional escape rhythm when the SA node fails to generate an impulse or if the rate of impulse generation falls below that of the AV node, then the AV node will assume the role of the pacemaker, the resulting rhythm is called a junctional escape rhythm

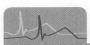

TABLE 9–2 Junctional escape rhythm

Questions 1–5	Answers
1. What is the rate?	Usually 40–60 BPM
2. What is the rhythm?	Usually regular; irregular if isolated junctional escape beat is present
3. Is there a P wave before each QRS? Are the P waves upright and uniform?	Inverted or absent May appear before or after the QRS
4. What is the length of the PR interval?	Usually less than 0.12 sec if P wave precedes QRS; absent if no P wave occurs before QRS
5. Do all the QRS complexes look alike? What is the Length of the QRS Complexes?	Yes Less than 0.12 sec (3 small squares)

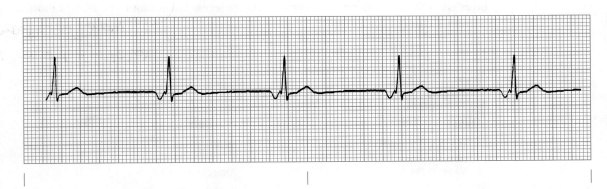

FIGURE 9–2. Junctional escape rhythm

In Figure 9–2, you should note the heart rate as 50 BPM, the rhythm is regular, P wave is inverted, the PRI is 0.12 seconds, and the QRS is 0.04 seconds. These findings should validate Junctional Escape Rhythm.

Remember that the rate of a junctional escape rhythm will be the intrinsic rate of the AV junctional tissue (40–60 BPM), and the P waves may be inverted or absent or may occur after the QRS complexes. **Remember . . . always monitor your patient's clinical condition!**

ACCELERATED JUNCTIONAL RHYTHMS

In our earlier discussion of the properties of the heart, we addressed the term automaticity. This term refers to the capability of the pacemaker cells of the heart to self-depolarize. Increased automaticity in the AV junction, causing the junction to discharge impulses at a rate faster than its intrinsic rate, results in a dysrhythmia referred to as **accelerated junctional rhythm**.

We generally refer to rhythms as tachycardic when the rate exceeds 100 BPM. In comparison with the intrinsic rate of the AV junction (40–60 BPM), the rate of this rhythm is generally around 60 to 100 BPM, thus the term *accelerated*. When the junctional firing rate is between 100 and 160 BPM, the resulting rhythm is called **junctional tachycardia**; we discuss this rhythm in the next section of this chapter. As you may now realize,

accelerated junctional rhythm increased automaticity in the AV junction, causing the junction to discharge impulses at a rate faster than its intrinsic rate

junctional tachycardia when the junctional firing rate exceeds 100 BPM

description of the junctional rhythms is, in part, specific to the rate of impulse generation from the AV junction.

Causes of accelerated junctional rhythms include ischemia of the AV junction, hypoxia, digitalis intoxication, inferior wall myocardial infarction, and rheumatic fever. As with any dysrhythmia, and especially if symptoms are present, the patient should be carefully monitored.

You should, at this time, ask and answer the five questions that apply to interpreting an EKG rhythm strip. (See ■ **Table 9–3** and ■ **Figure 9–3**.) Remember to apply each question slowly and methodically to the strip that you are observing in order to gain a complete understanding of the interpretation of the rhythm. Remember that memorization of strips *does not work* and will often lead you down the path to incorrect analysis. If in doubt, start over and ask the five questions again.

In Figure 9–3, you should note the heart rate as 70 BPM, the rhythm is regular, P wave is absent, the PRI is absent, and the QRS is 0.08 seconds. These findings should validate Accelerated Junctional Rhythm.

Remember that the rate of an accelerated junctional rhythm (60–100 BPM) will be greater than the intrinsic rate of the AV junction (40–60 BPM), and the P waves may be inverted or absent or occur after the QRS complexes. **Remember . . . always monitor your patient's clinical condition!**

If more escalautes 101→ JUCtional tachcardi.

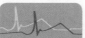

TABLE 9–3 Accelerated junctional rhythm

Questions 1–5	Answers
1. What is the rate?	60–100 BPM
2. What is the rhythm?	Atrial: regular Ventricular: regular
3. Is there a P wave before each QRS? Are the P waves upright and uniform?	Inverted or absent May appear before or after the QRS
4. What is the length of the PR interval?	Usually less than 0.12 sec if P wave precedes QRS; absent if no P wave occurs before QRS
5. Do all the QRS complexes look alike? What is the length of the QRS complexes?	Yes Less than 0.12 sec (3 small squares)

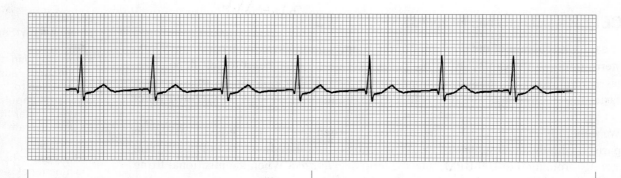

FIGURE 9–3. Accelerated junctional rhythm

JUNCTIONAL TACHYCARDIA RHYTHMS

In our discussion of accelerated junctional rhythm, we determined that increased automaticity in the AV junction may cause the pacemaker cells of the junction to discharge impulses at a rate faster than its intrinsic rate. We also noted that rates exceeding 100 BPM are referred to as tachycardic. Assimilating these two facts, we now recognize that a rhythm arising from the AV junctional tissue at a rate of 100 to 180 BPM is referred to as a **junctional tachycardia rhythm**. Junctional tachycardias are rare, but are seen occasionally among patients with SVT (supraventricular tachycardia).

In our discussion of the atrial rhythms (Chapter 8), we determined that a rhythm observed to start or end abruptly is referred to as a **paroxysmal rhythm**. Thus a junctional tachycardia rhythm that is *observed* to begin or end abruptly is correctly called a **paroxysmal junctional tachycardia (PJT) rhythm**. Due to the rapid rate of a paroxysmal junctional tachycardia rhythm, it may be indistinguishable from other supraventricular tachycardic rhythms. Consequently, PJT may simply, and correctly, be referred to as a PSVT rhythm.

Causes of junctional tachycardia rhythms may include underlying ischemic heart disease, frequent ingestion of stimulants, anxiety, hypoxia, medications such as digitalis, rheumatic heart disease, or may be idiopathic in nature. An interesting aspect of PJT is that this rhythm may occur at any age, in a patient with no history of underlying cardiac disease. As with other dysrhythmias, treatment (if indicated) is aimed at identifying and treating the underlying cause of the dysrhythmia.

Let's now apply the five-step approach to rhythm analysis to understand junctional tachycardia. (See ■ **Table 9–4** and ■ **Figure 9–4**.)

junctional tachycardia rhythm rhythm arising from the AV junctional tissue at a rate of 100 to 180 BPM

paroxysmal rhythm rhythm observed to start or end abruptly

paroxysmal junctional tachycardia (PJT) rhythm a junctional tachycardia rhythm that is observed to begin or end abruptly

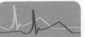

TABLE 9–4 Junctional tachycardia

Questions 1–5	Answers
1. What is the rate?	100–180 BPM
2. What is the rhythm?	Atrial: regular Ventricular: regular
3. Is there a P wave before each QRS? Are the P waves upright and uniform?	If visible, inverted May appear before or after the QRS
4. What is the length of the PR interval?	Usually less than 0.12 sec if P wave precedes QRS; absent if no P wave occurs before QRS
5. Do all the QRS complexes look alike? What is the length of the QRS complexes?	Yes Less than 0.12 sec (3 small squares)

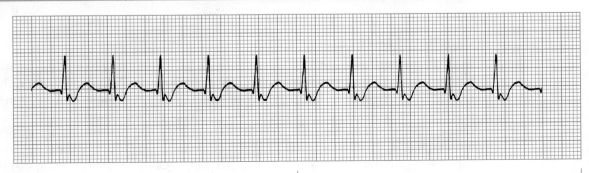

FIGURE 9–4. Junctional tachycardia rhythm

In Figure 9–4, you should note the heart rate as 100 BPM, the rhythm is regular, P wave appears after the QRS and is upright, the PRI is absent, and the QRS is 0.04 seconds. These findings should validate Junctional Tachycardia Rhythm.

Remember that the rate of a junctional tachycardia rhythm will be greater than 100 BPM. The P waves may be inverted (if visible) or absent or may occur after the QRS complexes. **Remember . . . always monitor your patient's clinical condition!**

CLINICAL SIGNIFICANCE OF JUNCTIONAL RHYTHMS

Premature junctional contractions

The clinical significance of PJCs is based on the frequency of their occurrence and, most importantly, on the patient's clinical condition. Normally, isolated PJCs are of minimal significance. If PJCs are frequent (more than 6 per minute), you should recognize that more serious dysrhythmias may develop. In addition, frequent PJCs may signify underlying organic heart disease. Typically, management of patients who present with isolated PJCs includes only close observation.

Junctional escape rhythm

The clinical significance of junctional escape rhythms is based on the patient's heart rate and clinical condition. We recall now that the intrinsic rate of the AV junctional tissue is 40 to 60 BPM. If the patient's heart rate is nearer the lower end of the range, it is wise to be concerned with the possibility of decreased cardiac output. Decreased cardiac output may precipitate angina.

Patients may exhibit signs and symptoms of decreased perfusion, such as altered mental status, dizziness, and decreased blood pressure (hypotension). Treatment may include the administration of oxygen, as well as the consideration of atropine administration (or treatment per local protocols). If however, the rate is nearer 50 to 60 BPM, the junctional escape rhythm may be well tolerated.

Accelerated junctional rhythm

Accelerated junctional rhythm is generally well tolerated by the patient and usually requires no immediate intervention. In dealing with patients who are taking the drug digoxin, accelerated junctional rhythm may suggest the possibility of digitalis toxicity. Because ischemia is one possible cause of this rhythm, the patient must be carefully monitored for the occurrence of other, more serious dysrhythmias.

Junctional tachycardia rhythm

In a young patient with a healthy heart, junctional tachycardia may be well tolerated. This is not the case, however, in patients with cardiac compromise. Patients may report that they feel as though the heart is running away or fluttering. Cardiac output may be significantly decreased due to inadequate ventricular filling time. Sustained episodes of junctional tachycardia, especially at the high-rate range (160–180 BPM), may precipitate angina, congestive heart failure, pronounced hypoxia, or hypotension. Treatment is based on the patient's clinical appearance, signs, and symptoms and may include vagal maneuvers, drug therapy, and electrical therapy.

CHAPTER 9

SUMMARY

Rhythms that are initiated in the area of the AV junction are called junctional rhythms. It will be helpful for you to recognize that all junctional dysrhythmias contain several similar EKG features. These common features include P waves that are inverted or absent, a PR interval that is usually less than 0.12 seconds in duration, and QRS complexes that are within normal limits. Typically, management of patients who present with junctional rhythms involves only close observation.

KEY POINTS TO REMEMBER

1. Junctional rhythms are those that initiate in the area of the AV junction.
2. Premature junctional contractions (PJCs) initiate from a single site in the AV junction and arise earlier than the next anticipated complex.
3. Noncompensatory pause occurs after an ectopic beat when the SA node is depolarizing, causing the underlying rhythm of the heart to be interrupted.
4. Compensatory pause occurs after an ectopic beat in which the SA node is unaffected and the underlying rhythm of the heart is not interrupted.
5. A junctional escape rhythm occurs when the SA node fails to generate an impulse or falls below the rate of the AV node; the AV node will assume the role of the pacemaker.
6. When the AV junction discharges impulses at a rate faster than its intrinsic rate, this rhythm is referred to as an accelerated junctional rhythm.
7. When the junctional firing rate exceeds 100 BPM, it is termed a junctional tachycardia.
8. A junctional tachycardia rhythm that is observed to begin or end abruptly is called a paroxysmal junctional tachycardia.
9. When an impulse travels in a retrograde direction, it is moving in a backward direction in the electrical conduction system.
10. The rate of accelerated junctional rhythm will be greater than the intrinsic firing rate of the AV junction.

REVIEW QUESTIONS

1. The AV node is located in the:
   a. Right atrium
   b. Left ventricle
   c. Purkinje fiber tract
   d. Intraventricular septum

2. The intrinsic firing rate of the AV node is _____ BPM.
   a. 15–25
   b. 25–35
   c. 35–45
   d. 40–60

3. The intrinsic rate of the SA node in an adult is
   _____ BPM.
   a. 20–60   c. 60–100
   b. 40–80   d. 80–100

4. The treatment of uncomplicated acute myocardial
   infarction usually includes:
   a. IV D5W, PCI
   b. Oxygen by mask, IV LR, PCI
   c. IV NS, monitor, O$_2$ via nasal cannula
   d. IV NS, monitor, O$_2$, PCI or fibrinolytic therapy

5. The chambers of the heart that are thin walled and
   pump against low pressure are the:
   a. Apex   c. Atria
   b. Aorta   d. Ventricles

6. To distinguish PJT from sinus tachycardia, recall
   that a usual EKG feature of PJT is a _____
   rate.
   a. More rapid   c. Less irregular
   b. Less rapid   d. More irregular

7. Rhythms that are _____ develop above the
   ventricles.
   a. Superventricular   c. Supraventricular
   b. Idioventricular   d. Retroventricular

8. PJCs resemble:
   a. PVCs   c. PACs
   b. PATs   d. PSVT

9. The rate of junctional tachycardia rhythms must be
   greater than _____ BPM.
   a. 200   c. 300
   b. 100   d. 260

10. When interpreting junctional rhythms, you should
    realize that the P waves may be:
    a. Inverted   c. Hidden in the QRS
    b. Absent   d. Any of the above

11. Premature junctional contractions (or complexes)
    are less common than premature atrial complexes
    (PACs) or premature ventricular contractions
    (PVCs).
    a. True   b. False

12. Causes of PJCs may include:
    a. Fever   c. Drug effects
    b. Anxiety   d. All the above

13. Myocardial ischemia can precipitate PJCs.
    a. True   b. False

14. PJCs may occur without any definite underlying
    cause.
    a. True   b. False

15. It is important to note that isolated occurrences of
    PJCs are not life-threatening.
    a. True   b. False

 REVIEW STRIPS

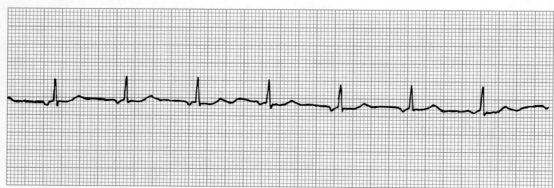

1. Rate _____   Rhythm _____

   P wave _____   PR interval _____

   QRS complex _____   Interpretation _____

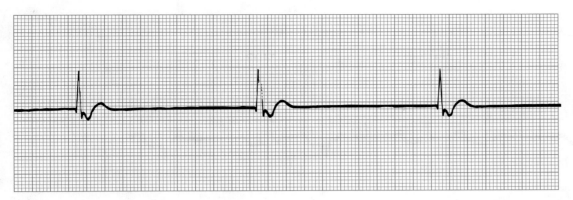

2. Rate _____   Rhythm _____

    P wave _____   PR interval _____

    QRS complex _____   Interpretation _____

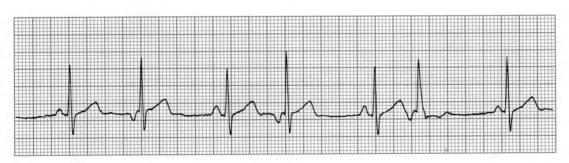

3. Rate _____   Rhythm _____

    P wave _____   PR interval _____

    QRS complex _____   Interpretation _____

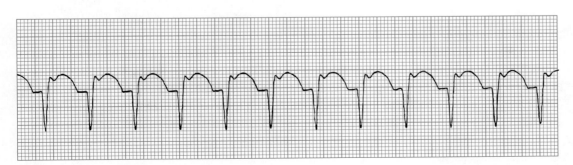

4. Rate _____   Rhythm _____

    P wave _____   PR interval _____

    QRS complex _____   Interpretation _____

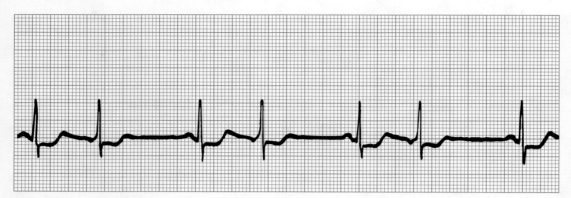

5. Rate _____   Rhythm _____
    P wave _____   PR interval _____
    QRS complex _____   Interpretation _____

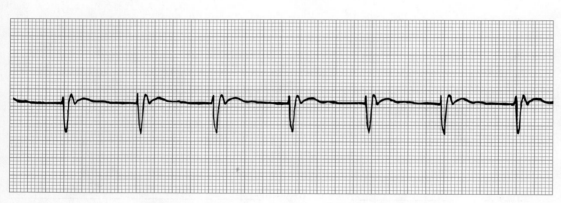

6. Rate _____   Rhythm _____
    P wave _____   PR interval _____
    QRS complex _____   Interpretation _____

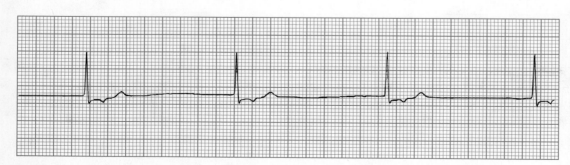

7. Rate _____   Rhythm _____
    P wave _____   PR interval _____
    QRS complex _____   Interpretation _____

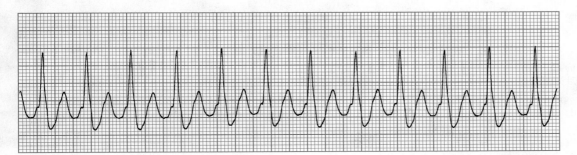

8. Rate _____   Rhythm _____

    P wave _____   PR interval _____

    QRS complex _____   Interpretation _____

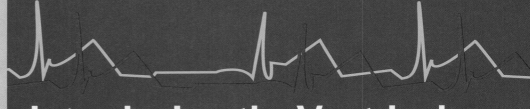

10

Objectives

Upon completion of this chapter, the student will be able to:

- Review specific components of the electrical conduction system of the heart
- Discuss the origin of the ventricular rhythms
- Identify premature ventricular contractions, including EKG characteristics
- Explain idioventricular rhythm, including EKG characteristics
- Differentiate idioventricular rhythm and accelerated idioventricular rhythm
- Distinguish ventricular tachycardia, including EKG characteristics
- Identify ventricular fibrillation, including EKG characteristics
- Recognize ventricular asystole, including EKG characteristics
- Discuss pulseless electrical activity
- Discuss the clinical significance of the ventricular rhythms

Introducing the Ventricular Rhythms

INTRODUCTION

In previous chapters, we have discussed rhythms that originate above the ventricles, or supraventricular rhythms. In this chapter, we will explore rhythms that have their origin in the ventricles. Ventricular rhythms are characteristically considered more dangerous than supraventricular rhythms. Despite this broad statement, it is imperative to remember that the significance of *any* rhythm is based on your patient's clinical condition.

REVIEW OF THE HEART'S ELECTRICAL CONDUCTION SYSTEM

In Chapter 8, we learned that the electrical activity produced by the conduction system of the heart is recorded as waveforms on EKG paper. Recall that the sinoatrial (SA) node is the usual, or expected, site of impulse generation. The electrical impulse leaves the SA node at a rate of 60 to 100 beats per minute (BPM) and travels through the atria via the internodal pathways, resulting in atrial depolarization. The atrioventricular (AV) node then receives and slows the impulse before allowing it to travel on through the AV junction, the bundle of His, and the left and right bundle branches, and down through the Purkinje fibers in the ventricles, causing ventricular depolarization. Although we know now that this is the normal route of impulses through the electrical conduction system, we have also learned that many variations can occur. One group of variations is called ventricular dysrhythmias.

ORIGIN OF VENTRICULAR RHYTHMS

Recall now that the pacemaker cells in the ventricles can, in certain instances, serve as the heart's pacemaker. An electrical impulse can be initiated from any pacemaker cell in the ventricles, including the bundle branches or the fibers of the Purkinje network.

When the SA node or the AV junctional tissues fail to initiate an electrical impulse, the ventricles will assume the responsibility of pacing the heart. Think now about the intrinsic firing rate of the three pacemaker sites and review ■ **Table 10–1**.

A brief review of this table clearly reminds you that the heart rate is significantly decreased when the ventricles assume the responsibility of pacing the heart. Remembering the relationship between heart rate and cardiac output immediately alerts us to the fact that cardiovascular compromise is a very real consideration when the ventricles are acting as the pacemaker of the heart. It is safe to say that the ventricles are the least efficient of the heart's pacemakers. This knowledge alone will alert us to the fact that the patient must be even more carefully monitored when the EKG strip or cardiac monitor demonstrates the attributes of a ventricular rhythm.

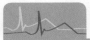

TABLE 10–1 Intrinsic firing rates of pacemaker sites

Sinoatrial (SA) node	60–100 BPM
Atrioventricular (AV) junctional tissue	40–60 BPM
Purkinje network	20–40 BPM

Impulses that are ventricular in origin begin in the lower ventricular musculature. Hence, the impulse may travel in a retrograde (backward) direction in order to depolarize the atria. Depending upon the actual *site of origin,* the impulse may travel antegrade (forward) to depolarize the ventricles. In either direction of travel, the normal conduction pathway is bypassed. Because of this bypass, ventricular rhythms display QRS complexes that are wide (greater than or equal to 0.12 sec) and bizarre in appearance, and P waves are absent. P waves are indistinguishable because they are buried or hidden in the QRS complex. Remember that the QRS complexes of supraventricular rhythms are commonly less than 0.12 seconds in duration.

PREMATURE VENTRICULAR COMPLEXES (CONTRACTIONS)

3/24/16
↳ somewher in the ventricle

In the initial discussion of premature ventricular complexes (PVCs), it is important to note that PVCs are individual complexes *rather than* an actual rhythm. In your future studies of premature beats, you will undoubtedly find references to premature beats as contractions rather than complexes. It is wise, however, to realize that the more correct term to be used in the discussion of these premature beats is complex, not contraction.

During a premature ventricular contraction, the ventricle electrically discharges (contracts) prematurely before the normal electrical impulses arrive from the SA node. These premature discharges are most commonly due to electrical "irritability" of the heart muscle of the ventricles and can be caused by a variety of issues, including, but not limited to myocardial infarction, electrolyte imbalances, oxygen deficits, or medications. Immediately after a premature ventricular contraction, the electrical system of the heart resets. This resetting causes a brief pause in the heartbeat, and some patients report feeling the heart briefly "stopping" after a premature ventricular contraction.

A single, ectopic (out-of-place) complex that occurs earlier than the next expected complex and arises from an irritable site in the ventricles is referred to as a **premature ventricular complex**. Premature ventricular complexes are quite common occurrences and can appear in many heart rhythms. The significance of the appearance of PVCs is based entirely upon the patient's clinical condition.

Most commonly, the underlying cadence of the SA node is not interrupted by the occurrence of a PVC, nor is the SA node depolarized by the PVC. A premature ventricular complex is usually followed by a compensatory pause. Recall our earlier discussions regarding compensatory and noncompensatory pauses. You will remember that a compensatory pause is one in which the SA node is unaffected, nor is the cadence of the heart interrupted. The presence of *a compensatory pause,* coupled with a wide, bizarre, and premature QRS complex, is a highly suggestive indicator of PVCs.

On occasion, a PVC may fall between two sinus beats without interfering with the rhythm. This beat is referred to as an **interpolated beat**. As you are about to learn, PVCs may appear in many different patterns and shapes. Perhaps it is because of their bizarre appearance that PVCs are usually easier to discern than other premature beats.

The **morphology**, or shape, of the PVC is based on the site of origin of the ectopic focus. PVCs that are alike in appearance are called **unifocal**, whereas those with different

premature ventricular complex single, ectopic (out-of-place) complex that occurs earlier than the next expected complex and arises from an irritable site in the ventricles

interpolated beat when a PVC falls between two sinus beats without interfering with the rhythm

morphology shape of the PVC

unifocal PVCs that are alike in appearance

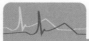

TABLE 10–2 PVC patterns of occurrence

Ventricular bigeminy	Occurs when every other beat is a PVC
Ventricular trigeminy	Occurs when every third beat is a PVC
Ventricular quadrigeminy	Occurs when every fourth beat is a PVC
Couplet or repetitive PVCs	Two PVCs occurring together without a normal complex in between
Runs of ventricular tachycardia (V tach)	Three or more PVCs in a row

multifocal PVCs with different shapes that originate from different sites within the ventricles

shapes are called **multifocal**. Unifocal PVCs arise from one single site within the ventricles, whereas multifocal PVCs originate from different sites within the ventricles. Because PVCs often indicate myocardial irritability, you should note that multifocal PVCs are more serious than unifocal PVCs. If, for instance, you note an EKG strip containing PVCs with three or four different shapes, it should occur to you that there may be three or four different irritable sites within the ventricles. Any indication of increased myocardial irritability dictates that the patient should be carefully evaluated and managed without delay. PVCs may be classified based on the basis of their frequency of occurrence, as illustrated in ■ **Table 10–2**.

We should note here that there should be at least three episodes in a row on the monitor or EKG strip in order to correctly identify patterns of ventricular bigeminy, trigeminy, or quadrigeminy. Another name given to a run or grouping of three or more PVCs in a row (ventricular tachycardia, or V tach, which is discussed later in this chapter) is **salvos**.

salvos another name given to a run or grouping of three or more PVCs in a row

Because the terms that identify patterns of occurrences of PVCs can also be applied to PACs and PJCs, it may be wise to note the site of origin when identifying premature beats. In other words, rather than simply stating *bigeminy,* a more correct interpretation might be *ventricular bigeminy*. Again, it's better to add a millisecond of time to your rhythm interpretation than to risk the possibility of an incorrect interpretation.

Test yourself by asking why ventricular bigeminy, couplets, and runs of ventricular tachycardia are very significant rhythm presentations. You should have answered the question by recalling that these particular rhythms tend to indicate increased myocardial irritability and may be precursors of more serious, perhaps lethal, dysrhythmias. This is even more notable if the PVCs happen to occur during the relative refractory, or vulnerable, period, during repolarization. Premature ventricular complexes are considered particularly dangerous if they occur more than six times in a 1-minute EKG strip (frequent PVCs), if they occur in couplets or runs of V tach, or if they occur in a patient who is hemodynamically unstable.

Premature ventricular complexes are also considered very dangerous if they fall on the T wave of the preceding beat (R-on-T phenomenon). If you recall our earlier discussion of the refractory periods, you will understand that the myocardium is in its most vulnerable state (electrically) during this period. A PVC that falls on the T wave may thus trigger repetitious ventricular contractions, resulting in ventricular fibrillation.

myocardial ischemia decreased supply of oxygenated blood to the heart

Causes of premature ventricular complexes include myocardial irritability (due to **myocardial ischemia**), increased emotional stress or physical exertion, congestive heart failure, electrolyte imbalances, digitalis toxicity, acid-base imbalances or blunt force trauma induced cardiac contusions. It is important to note that PVCs may also occur as simply a normal variant in some individuals. A PVC may be perceived by the patient as a "skipped" beat or felt as a palpitation in the chest. Treatment of PVCs, as with all dysrhythmias, is based on the patient's clinical symptoms and may range from the administration of oxygen to pharmaceutical antidysrhythmics.

Let's now apply the five-step approach to investigate the rules for interpretation of PVCs. (See ■ **Table 10–3** and ■ **Figures 10–1** through **10–6**.)

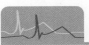 **TABLE 10–3 Premature ventricular complexes**

Questions 1–5	Answers
1. What is the rate?	Dependent on rate of underlying rhythm and number of PVCs
2. What is the rhythm?	Occasionally irregular; regular if interpolated PVC
3. Is there a P wave before each QRS?	No P waves associated with PVC
Are the P waves upright and uniform?	P waves of underlying rhythm may be present
4. What is the length of the PR interval?	PRI not present with PVCs
5. What do the QRS complexes look like?	Usually wide and bizarre
What is the length of the QRS complexes?	Equal to or greater than 0.12 sec (3 small squares)

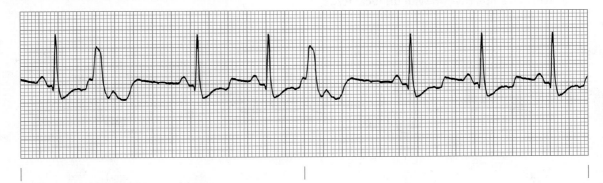

FIGURE 10–1. Compensatory pause following PVCs

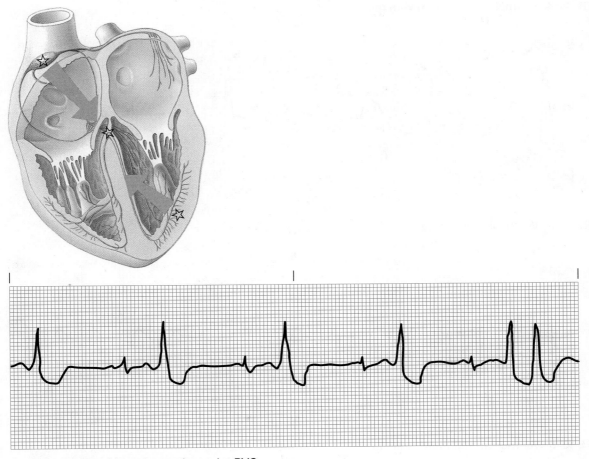

FIGURE 10–2. Ventricular bigeminy and couplet PVCs

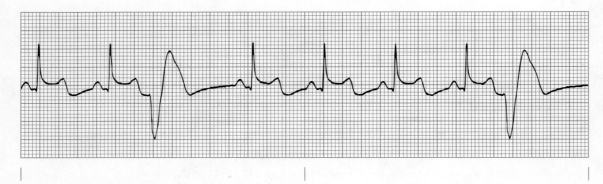

FIGURE 10–3. Normal sinus rhythm with unifocal PVCs

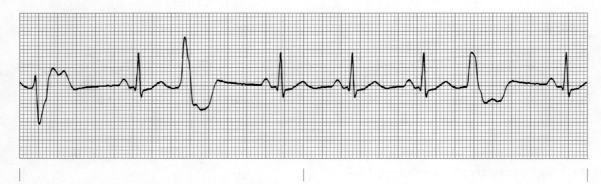

FIGURE 10–4. Normal sinus rhythm with multifocal PVCs

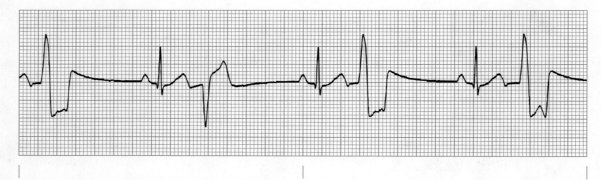

FIGURE 10–5. Ventricular bigeminy

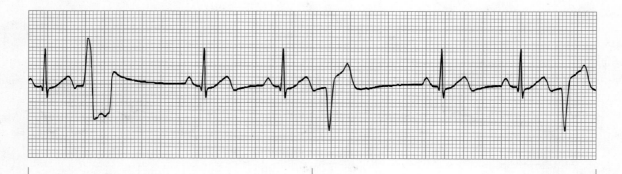

FIGURE 10–6. Ventricular trigeminy

In Figure 10–1, you should note the heart rate as 80 BPM, the rhythm is irregular, P wave is present and upright in normal complexes, the PRI is 0.16 seconds in normal complexes, and the QRS is 0.04 seconds in normal complexes. These findings should validate Compensatory Pause following PVCs.

In Figure 10–2, you should note the heart rate as 60 BPM, the rhythm is irregular, P wave is present and upright in normal complexes, the PRI is 0.12 seconds in normal complexes, and the QRS is 0.04 seconds in normal complexes. These findings should validate Ventricular Bigeminy and Couplet PVCs.

In Figure 10–3, you should note the heart rate as 80 BPM, the rhythm is irregular, P wave is present and upright in normal complexes, the PRI is 0.16 seconds in normal complexes, and the QRS is 0.04 seconds in normal complexes. These findings should validate Sinus Rhythm with PVCs.

In Figure 10–4, you should note the heart rate as 80 BPM, the rhythm is irregular, P wave is present and upright in normal complexes, the PRI is 0.16 seconds in normal complexes, and the QRS is 0.06 seconds in normal complexes. These findings should validate Sinus Rhythm with Multifocal PVCs.

In Figure 10–5, you should note the heart rate as 70 BPM, the rhythm is irregular, P wave is present and upright in normal complexes, the PRI is 0.16 seconds in normal complexes, and the QRS is 0.04 seconds in normal complexes. These findings should validate Ventricular Bigeminy.

In Figure 10–6, you should note the heart rate as 80 BPM, the rhythm is irregular, P wave is present and upright in normal complexes, the PRI is 0.16 seconds in normal complexes, and the QRS is 0.04 seconds. These findings should validate Ventricular Trigeminy.

Remember that the number of PVCs is included in the total count of R waves in calculating the rate in rhythms containing PVCs. One key in the recognition of PVCs is the usual wide, bizarre appearance of the QRS. **Remember . . . always monitor your patient's clinical condition!**

IDIOVENTRICULAR RHYTHM

Idioventricular rhythms (IVRs) are also called *ventricular escape rhythms* and are considered a last-ditch effort of the ventricles to try to prevent cardiac standstill. The appearance of this rhythm most commonly indicates that the SA node and the AV junctional tissue have failed to function as pacemakers or that the rate of these higher pacemakers has fallen below the intrinsic rate of the ventricles. Neither P waves nor PR intervals (PRIs) are produced because the atria do not depolarize. Although ventricular depolarization does occur, the rate is usually less than 40 BPM and cardiac output is usually compromised.

When the rate of an IVR rhythm falls below 20 BPM, the rhythm may be called **agonal**. Agonal rhythm may frequently be seen as the last ordered semblance of heart rhythm when a resuscitation attempt has been unsuccessful. IVR may commonly be seen as the first organized rhythm following successful defibrillation. Causes of IVR include extensive myocardial damage, secondary to acute myocardial infarction, or failure of higher pacemakers. IVR usually results in symptoms related to decreased cardiac output (hypotension, cool & clammy skin, dizziness, syncope, chest pain, and dyspnea). IVR is, in most cases, considered a lethal rhythm, and treatment must be immediate and aggressive. Based on the patient's heart rate, the treatment may follow the same regimen as would be followed with symptomatic bradycardia, that is, oxygen, intravenous (IV) access, atropine IV push, as well as consideration of epinephrine and dopamine infusion, while preparing for possible transcutaneous pacing (TCP). As always, you should follow your local protocols.

idioventricular rhythms (IVRs) (also called ventricular escape rhythms) result when the discharge rate of higher pacemakers becomes less than that of the ventricles or when impulses from higher pacemakers fail to reach the ventricles

agonal when the rate of an IVR rhythm falls below 20 BPM, the rhythm may be called agonal

TABLE 10–4 Idioventricular rhythm

Questions 1–5	Answers
1. What is the rate?	20–40 BPM or less
2. What is the rhythm?	Atrial rhythm not distinguishable; ventricular rhythm usually regular
3. Is there a P wave before each QRS?	No; none present
4. What is the length of the PR interval?	None
5. Do all the QRS complexes look alike? What is the length of the QRS complexes?	Yes; bizarre morphology Greater than 0.12 sec

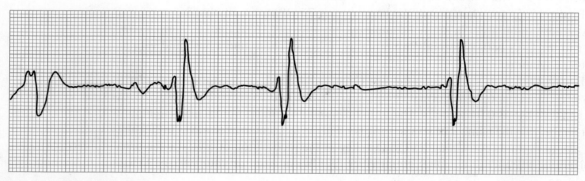

FIGURE 10–7. Idioventricular rhythm

Although the absence of P waves and the widened QRS complexes on the EKG strip are obvious, it is wise to follow your basic five-step approach in the interpretation of this rhythm. (See ■ **Table 10–4** and ■ **Figure 10–7**.)

Recognize that an idioventricular rhythm is an ominous sign. **It is critical that you remember to monitor your patient's clinical condition closely.**

ACCELERATED IDIOVENTRICULAR RHYTHM

accelerated idioventricular rhythm (AIVR) occurs when the rate of the ectopic pacemaker in an idioventricular rhythm exceeds 40 BPM

An **accelerated idioventricular rhythm (AIVR)** may occur when the rate of the ectopic pacemaker in an idioventricular rhythm exceeds 40 BPM. The commonly accepted rate of AIVR is 40 to 100 BPM. Because the atria do not depolarize, there are no P waves or PR intervals noted on an EKG strip that depicts AIVR. (See ■ **Figure 10–8**.)

In Figure 10–8, you should note the heart rate as 60 BPM, the rhythm is regular, P wave is absent, the PRI is absent, and the QRS is 0.16 seconds. These findings should validate Accelerated Idioventricular Rhythm.

AIVR may occur in conjunction with myocardial ischemia. Because of the morphology of the QRS complexes in ventricular dysrhythmias, it is very important that the heart rate be carefully evaluated. AIVR can be mistaken for ventricular tachycardia unless there is a careful assessment of the patient and the patient's heart rate. As noted earlier, the usual rate of an AIVR is 40 to 100 BPM; the rate of ventricular tachycardia is usually greater than 120 BPM.

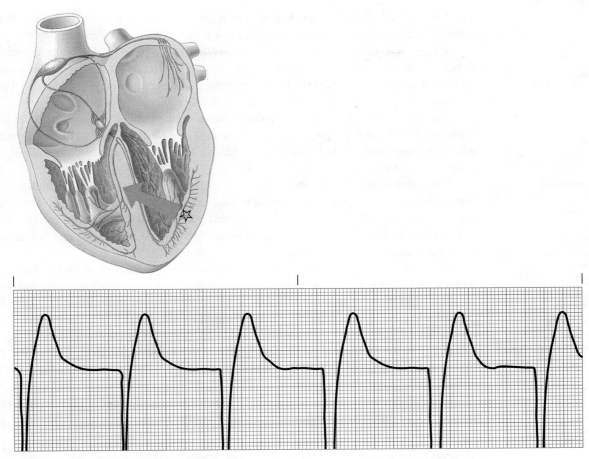

FIGURE 10–8. Accelerated idioventricular rhythm

AIVR is often the most common reperfusion dysrhythmia; however, Ventricular Tachycardia and Ventricular Fibrillation remain the most common causes of sudden death following spontaneous reperfusion. Although experts and various references may disagree on **exact** ranges of heart rates of ventricular dysrhythmias, it is imperative to *remember that you must always assess and treat the patient instead of the monitor or EKG strip.*

VENTRICULAR TACHYCARDIA 3/24/16

The most commonly accepted definition of **ventricular tachycardia (VT or V tach)** describes this rhythm as one in which three or more PVCs arise in sequence at a rate of greater than 100 BPM. This rhythm commonly overrides the normal pacemaker of the heart.

Quite often, this dysrhythmia occurs rapidly and is initiated by a PVC or by PVCs occurring in rapid succession. If this rhythm is sustained, the patient's clinical condition may rapidly deteriorate. It is important to note that some patients may, in fact, tolerate a sustained V tach rhythm without immediate decompensation; however, this is the exception, not the rule. A **sustained rhythm** is generally thought to be a rhythm that lasts for more than 30 seconds. If a run of VT lasts for less than 30 seconds, it is a **nonsustained rhythm**, or simply a run of V tach.

When a ventricular ectopic beat occurs at a rate of 100 to 250 BPM, V tach may result. P waves may be present if the SA node retains control of the atria; however, if P waves are present, they have no set relationship to the QRS complexes. PR intervals are not discernible.

ventricular tachycardia (VT, V tach) rhythm in which three or more PVCs arise in sequence at a rate of greater than 100 BPM; commonly overrides the normal pacemaker of the heart

sustained rhythm a rhythm that lasts for more than 30 seconds

nonsustained rhythm a run of V tach that lasts for less than 30 seconds

The QRS complexes in V tach will appear wide and bizarre, measuring greater than 0.12 seconds in duration. The ventricular rhythm in V tach is essentially regular.

V tach is classified (on the basis of assessment of the patients' clinical presentation) as either *pulseless V tach* or *V tach with a pulse*. Immediate treatment for the patient who exhibits V tach on the monitor is based on the presence or absence of a palpable pulse. Pulseless V tach is treated as ventricular fibrillation, with immediate defibrillation.

The treatment of V tach with a pulse is based on the patient's clinical picture; thus you must assess whether the patient is stable or unstable. If the patient is hemodynamically unstable, immediate cardioversion is considered. If the patient is hemodynamically stable, drug intervention is appropriate.

Hemodynamically unstable refers to a patient who presents with hypotension (low blood pressure), chest pain, shortness of breath, and changes in mental status. The change in mental status may signal a decrease in cerebral perfusion. A patient who is **hemodynamically stable** will usually present with a normal blood pressure (normotensive), absence of chest pain, and no notable change in mental status.

Causes of V tach are somewhat synonymous with the causes of PVCs. These causes include myocardial ischemia, hypoxia, electrolyte imbalances, cardiomegaly, myocarditis, valvular heart disease, increased anxiety or physical exertion, and underlying heart disease. Consider the key points regarding interpretation of V tach as you perform your five-step approach to the rhythm represented in ■ **Table 10–5** and ■ **Figure 10–9**.

In Figure 10–9, you should note the heart rate as 180 BPM, the rhythm is regular, P wave is absent, the PRI is absent, and the QRS is greater than 0.12 seconds. These findings should validate Ventricular Tachycardia.

Remember that V tach is a potentially life-threatening dysrhythmia. It is vital that you **remember to monitor your patient's clinical condition closely**.

TORSADES DE POINTES

A rhythm that is similar to V tach is **torsades de pointes**. This name is derived from a French term meaning "twisting of the points." The morphology of QRS complexes in a torsades rhythm shows variations in width and shape. This rhythm resembles a turning about or a twisting motion along the baseline (isoelectric line). Torsades is most often triggered by early premature ventricular contractions (R on T phenomenon). This life-threatening dys-

hemodynamically unstable refers to a patient who presents with hypotension (low blood pressure), chest pain, shortness of breath, and changes in mental status

hemodynamically stable refers to a patient who presents with a normal blood pressure (normotensive), absence of chest pain, and no notable change in mental status

torsades de pointes similar to ventricular tachycardia; morphology of QRS complexes show variations in width and shape; life-threatening dysrhythmia

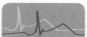

TABLE 10–5 Ventricular tachycardia rhythm

Questions 1–5	Answers
1. What is the rate?	100–250 BPM
2. What is the rhythm?	Atrial rhythm not distinguishable; ventricular rhythm usually regular
3. Is there a P wave before each QRS?	May be present or absent; not associated with QRS complexes
4. What is the length of the PR interval?	None
5. Do all the QRS complexes look alike? What is the length of the QRS complexes?	Yes (except in torsades rhythm); bizarre QRS morphology Greater than 0.12 sec

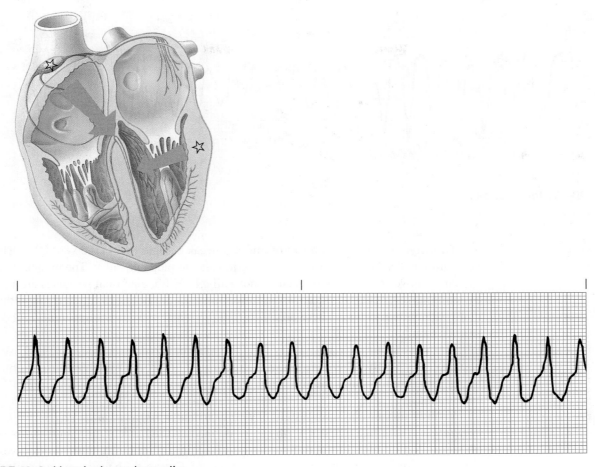

FIGURE 10–9. Ventricular tachycardia

rhythmia may result from hypokalemia, hypomagnesemia, an overdose of a tricyclic antidepressant drug, the use of antidysrhythmic drugs, or a combination of these.

Although torsades is often responsive to electrical therapy, it is wise to remember that this dysrhythmia has an annoying tendency to recur repeatedly. Therefore, finding and treating the underlying cause of the rhythm is essential. Magnesium is the pharmacologic treatment of choice for torsades de pointes. Some factors that are associated with an increased tendency toward torsades include hypocalcemia, hypoxia, acidosis, heart failure, and being female in gender. Treatment is directed toward withdrawal of offending agents, infusion of Magnesium Sulfate, antidysrhythmic drugs, and electrical therapy, as appropriate.

In ■ **Figure 10–10**, you should note the heart rate as 220 BPM, the rhythm is irregular, P wave is absent, the PRI is absent, and the QRS is greater than 0.12 seconds and appears to "twist" at the baseline. These findings should validate Torsades de Pointes.

Remember that the **key** to recognizing torsades is the variation of QRS morphology, or shape, as illustrated in Figure 10–10.

3/24/16

VENTRICULAR FIBRILLATION

Ventricular fibrillation (VF, V fib) is a fatal dysrhythmia, if not treated soon after onset. V fib is thought to be the most frequent initial rhythm occurrence in sudden cardiac arrest, according to the American Heart Association. V fib tends to occur in the initial hours following an acute myocardial infarction.

ventricular fibrillation (VF, V fib) is a fatal dysrhythmia that occurs as a result of multiple weak ectopic foci in the ventricles; there is no coordinated atrial or ventricular contraction and no palpable pulse

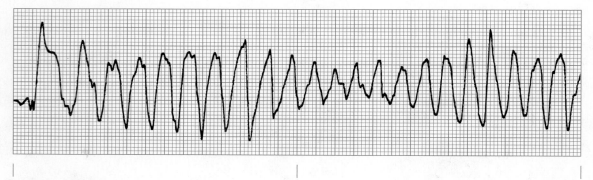

FIGURE 10–10. Torsades de pointes

This rhythm occurs as a result of multiple weak ectopic foci in the ventricles. There is no coordinated atrial or ventricular contraction and no palpable pulse. The myocardial cells appear to quiver rather than depolarize normally. In V fib, electrical impulses are initiated by multiple ventricular sites; however, these impulses are not transmitted through the normal conduction pathway. There are, therefore, no usual waveforms apparent on the EKG strip or monitor.

The waveforms in V fib appear as disorganized, rapid, irregular waves whose morphology vary vastly. There are no well-organized QRS complexes. Because no blood is being circulated throughout the body, death will occur if immediate treatment is not established.

V fib is further classified as either *fine ventricular fibrillation or coarse ventricular fibrillation.* These two types of V fib can be defined on the basis of amplitude (height) of V fib waves. V fib waves less than 3 mm in amplitude are described as *fine.* V fib waves with amplitudes greater than 3 mm are considered *coarse.* Coarse V fib waves are generally more irregular than fine V fib waves. Coarse V fib will progress to fine V fib unless treatment is initiated in a timely manner. It is notable to add that coarse V fib responds better than fine V fib to treatment (electrical therapy).

Thorough patient assessment is critical because artifact or loose leads can closely resemble ventricular fibrillation. Look at your patient and always, always *treat the patient, not the monitor.* If your patient is sitting up in bed, reading a newspaper, or conversing with you in a coherent manner, chances are *very good* that he or she is not experiencing V fib!

Causes of V fib include acute myocardial infarction, myocardial ischemia, drug toxicity or overdose, hypoxia, coronary artery disease, cardiomyopathy and a variety of other causes. Regardless of the cause of V fib, prompt intervention is vital to the survival of your patient.

As you review ■ **Table 10–6** and ■ **Figure 10–11** while applying the five-step approach, you may realize that the absence of waveforms indicates the absence of life-sustaining myocardial function.

Remember that V fib is a life-threatening dysrhythmia that will result in death unless immediate treatment is initiated. **Monitor your patient's clinical condition closely.**

In Figure 10–11, top-most strip, you should note the heart rate as indiscernible, the rhythm is irregular, P wave is absent, the PRI is absent and the QRS is indiscernible, fibrillatory waveforms are fine in nature. These findings should validate Fine Ventricular Fibrillation.

In Figure 10–11, bottom-most strip, you should note the heart rate as indiscernible, the rhythm is irregular, P wave is absent, the PRI is absent, and the QRS is indiscernible and appears coarse in nature. These findings should validate coarse Ventricular Fibrillation.

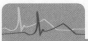 **TABLE 10–6 Ventricular fibrillation**

Questions 1–5	Answers
1. What is the rate?	Rate cannot be discerned
2. What is the rhythm?	Rapid, unorganized; rhythm not distinguishable
3. Is there a P wave before each QRS?	No
4. What is the length of the PR interval?	None present
5. Do all the QRS complexes look alike? What is the length of the QRS complexes?	None present

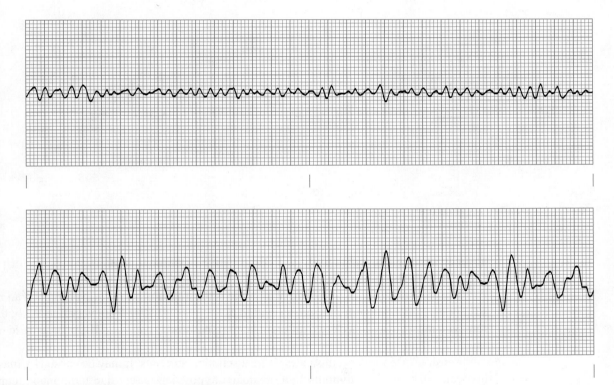

FIGURE 10–11. Ventricular fibrillation (fine and coarse)

Remember that V fib is a life-threatening dysrhythmia that will result in death unless immediate treatment is initiated. **Monitor your patient's clinical condition closely.**

ASYSTOLE OR VENTRICULAR ASYSTOLE   3/24/16

The absence of all ventricular activity is known as **ventricular asystole**. Ventricular asystole is also called **cardiac standstill**, or **asystole**. The technical, or literal, definition of asystole is the absence of all cardiac electrical activity. However, the terms are sometimes used interchangeably. Asystole is represented by a flat line (consistent with the isoelectric line on an EKG strip). Actually, asystole is not a rhythm; it represents the

ventricular asystole the absence of all ventricular activity; also called cardiac standstill or asystole; the absence of all cardiac electrical activity

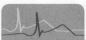 **TABLE 10–7 Ventricular asystole**

Questions 1–5	Answers
1. What is the rate?	Absent
2. What is the rhythm?	Absent; rhythm not distinguishable
3. Is there a P wave before each QRS?	No
4. What is the length of the PR interval?	None present
5. Do all the QRS complexes look alike? What is the length of the QRS complexes?	None present

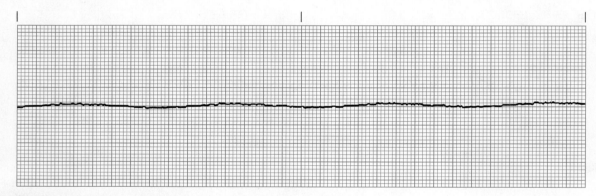

FIGURE 10–12. Ventricular asystole (cardiac standstill, asystole)

absence of all electrical activity and is indicative of clinical death (the absence of pulse and respirations).

The most notable characteristic of asystole is the total absence of waveforms on an EKG strip or cardiac monitor. It may be difficult to distinguish asystole from very fine V fib; therefore, you must always check two different leads (e.g., Lead II and Lead III) in order to identify asystole definitively.

Asystole often follows unsuccessful resuscitation attempts. It may be caused by massive myocardial infarction, hypothermia, acidosis, hypovolemia, cardiac tamponade, cardiac trauma, tension pneumothorax, ventricular aneurysm, and complete heart block. Ventricular asystole may often be the initial event in cardiac arrest.

In your application of the five-step approach to dysrhythmia interpretation, you will note that the rhythm in ■ **Table 10–7** and ■ **Figure 10–12** indicates the absence of both mechanical and electrical cardiac activity.

In Figure 10–12, you should note the heart rate as absent, the rhythm is not distinguishable, P wave is absent, the PRI is absent, and the QRS complex is absent. These findings should validate Asystole.

Resuscitation attempts are often unsuccessful, and the prognosis for patients who present with asystole is poor. Ventricular asystole is a terminal dysrhythmia and will result in death unless immediate treatment is initiated. **Closely monitor the patient's clinical condition!**

PULSELESS ELECTRICAL ACTIVITY 3/24/16

The absence of a palpable pulse and myocardial muscle activity with the presence of organized electrical activity (excluding V tach or V fib) on the cardiac monitor is called **pulseless electrical activity (PEA)**. There is electrical activity but the heart either does not contract or there are other reasons why this results in insufficient or no cardiac output. Pulseless electrical activity is not an actual rhythm; rather, it represents a clinical condition wherein the patient is clinically dead, despite the fact that some type of organized rhythm appears on the monitor. PEA was formerly called electromechanical dissociation (EMD). Like asystole, this rhythm conveys a grave prognosis.

Causes of PEA include profound hypovolemia, hypothermia, hyperthermia, drug overdose, hypokalemia, hyperkalemia, massive myocardial damage, ventricular rupture, pulmonary embolism, acidosis, and massive cardiac trauma, which may result in cardiac tamponade or tension pneumothorax. The underlying cause or causes of PEA must be rapidly identified and treated in order for the patient to survive. Treatment may include an IV fluid bolus, epinephrine and/or sodium bicarbonate.

pulseless electrical activity (PEA) absence of a palpable pulse and myocardial muscle activity with the presence of organized electrical activity (excluding V tach or V fib) on the cardiac monitor

CLINICAL SIGNIFICANCE OF VENTRICULAR DYSRHYTHMIAS

Premature ventricular complexes

Premature ventricular complexes may be of little or no significance in patients who have no history of heart disease. These patients may report a feeling of "skipped beats," and some patients will refer to the extra beats as **palpitations**. Patients may even relate that their intake of caffeine or their level of stress has increased recently. From previous experience, patients will often report that the skipped beats seemed to disappear when they reduced their intake of stimulants or their level of stress. This seems a good time to remind you that listening, *truly listening,* to your patients can be one of the most valuable assessment tools available to you.

palpitations sensation that the heart is skipping beats and/or beating rapidly

If your patient presents with evidence of myocardial ischemia (chest pain, anxiety, shortness of breath) and is exhibiting PVCs on the monitor or EKG strip, your index of suspicion should be heightened. Recall now that PVCs can indicate varying degrees of ventricular irritability and may be followed by more serious dysrhythmias. In addition, it is wise to remember that cardiac output may be compromised if PVCs are frequent. Recall the patterns of PVCs that are considered dangerous, or warning signs, and be alert for the occurrence of these patterns. Keep in mind that, often, the administration of oxygen may abate the PVCs. Most important, assess your patient's overall clinical picture. *Treat the patient, not the monitor!*

Idioventricular rhythm

The majority of patients who present with an idioventricular rhythm will be symptomatic. This is more easily understood when you recall that the heart rate is often slowed significantly with idioventricular rhythms. Cardiac compromise is always a concern in a patient with a slow heart rate. As a direct result of the decreased heart rate (bradycardia) and in conjunction with a decrease in cardiac output, the patient may present with weakness, dizziness, severe hypotension, and alterations in mental status.

It is essential that a thorough patient assessment be conducted in order to determine whether the rhythm is perfusing (producing a palpable pulse) or nonperfusing (signifying pulseless electrical activity). In instances of accelerated idioventricular rhythm, treatment is not indicated unless the patient is symptomatic. If the patient is symptomatic, the rhythm usually requires ventricular pacing as well as drug therapy including epinephrine, dopamine, and other pressor drugs to increase ventricular rate and support blood pressure.

3/24/16

Ventricular tachycardia

Ventricular tachycardia may be perfusing (producing a palpable pulse) or nonperfusing (producing no palpable pulse). Because of the rapid heart rate in V tach, the ventricles do not have time to adequately empty and refill; thus cardiac output will be compromised.

Recall that cardiac compromise can lead to decreased cerebral and myocardial perfusion because of inadequate amounts of blood circulating through the body. Treatment of V tach is based on the absence or presence of a palpable pulse, as well as the patient's clinical picture.

If the patient in V tach is perfusing and stable, treatment may consist of oxygen administration, implementation of an IV lifeline, and pharmacologic intervention. If the patient is (or becomes), clinically unstable (as evidenced by marked hypotension, chest pain, and shortness of breath), synchronized **cardioversion** may be indicated. If the patient is unstable (nonperfusing), the immediate treatment will consist of unsynchronized cardioversion (**defibrillation**). Remember that pulseless V tach is treated as if it were V fib. The treatment must be aggressive and immediate.

3/24/16

Ventricular fibrillation

With V fib, there is no cardiac output, no perfusion, and no evidence of organized electrical activity in the heart. In other words, the patient is in cardiac arrest. If this rhythm is not treated immediately and aggressively, the patient will not be able to sustain life. Most cardiac arrests result from either V tach or V fib. The presence of fine V fib indicates that the rhythm has been present for an extended period of time. Treatment for V fib must be immediate and decisive. This treatment includes CPR, defibrillation (360 joules [J], deliver one shock using monophasic or equivalent biphasic wave forms), airway control, IV lifeline or IO access, and drug intervention.

Most health care providers now use biphasic defibrillators. The recommended therapy is 120 to 200 joules as the initial dose; second and subsequent doses should be equivalent and higher doses should be considered.

The prognosis for patients with this life-threatening rhythm is less than encouraging. Nevertheless, the patient is treated aggressively in order to give him or her every possible chance to survive.

3/24/16

Asystole

Ventricular asystole signals a complete termination of ventricular activity. Often asystole is considered a confirmation of death. Always remember to check the rhythm in two leads in order to rule out the possibility of the presence of fine V fib. If the rhythm appears to be fine V fib, it should be treated as V fib. Treatment of asystole, if attempted, includes CPR, placement of IV lifelines, endotracheal intubation, and pharmacologic intervention. Contrary to many popular television programs, defibrillation is not indicated with asystole! As with *all* dysrhythmias, treatment must always be based on conscientious and thorough patient assessment.

cardioversion refers to the process of the passage of an electric current through the heart during a specific part of the cardiac cycle for the purpose of terminating certain kinds of dysrhythmias

defibrillation the process of passing an electrical current through a fibrillating heart to depolarize the cells and allow them to repolarize uniformly, thus restoring an organized/normal rhythm after the onset of fibrillation

CHAPTER 10

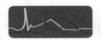 SUMMARY

The group of rhythms discussed in this chapter comprise the rhythms that are most commonly considered life-threatening. Ventricular rhythms often indicate myocardial ischemia and consequently must be diligently assessed and, where indicated, treated aggressively. In many instances, the outcome for the patient may depend upon the rapidity of recognition and treatment of ventricular dysrhythmias.

 KEY POINTS TO REMEMBER

1. When the SA node or the AV junctional tissues fail to initiate an electrical impulse, the ventricles will take the responsibility of pacing the heart.

2. It is important to note that PVCs are individual complexes *rather than* an actual rhythm.

3. Unifocal PVCs are similar in appearance, whereas multifocal PVCs originate from different sites within the ventricles and present with different morphology.

4. PVC patterns of occurrence include ventricular bigeminy, ventricular trigeminy, ventricular quadrigeminy, couplet or repetitive PVCs, and runs of ventricular tachycardia (V tach).

5. The appearance of an idioventricular ventricular rhythm commonly indicates that the SA node and the AV junctional tissue have failed to function as pacemakers or that the rate of these higher pacemakers has fallen below the intrinsic rate of the ventricles.

6. A ventricular tachycardia (VT or V tach) rhythm is described as one in which three or more PVCs arise in sequence at a rate of greater than 100 BPM.

7. Torsades de pointes rhythm resembles a turning about or a twisting motion along the baseline (isoelectric line).

8. Ventricular fibrillation (VF or V fib) is thought to be the most frequent initial rhythm occurrence in sudden cardiac arrest.

9. Asystole is represented by a flat line (consistent with the isoelectric line on an EKG strip) and represents no electrical activity in the heart.

10. Pulseless electrical activity (PEA) is not an actual rhythm; rather, it represents a clinical condition wherein the patient is clinically dead, despite the fact that some type of organized rhythm appears on the monitor.

 REVIEW QUESTIONS

1. PVCs characteristically have a _____ pause.
   a. Noncompensatory
   b. Uncompensatory
   c. Compensatory
   d. 0.30-seconds

2. The QRS complex corresponds to what electrical activity in the heart?
   a. Ventricular depolarization
   b. Atrial depolarization
   c. Ventricular contraction
   d. Atrial contraction

3. Pacemaker cells found in the Purkinje network in the ventricles have an intrinsic firing rate of _____ BPM.
   a. 20–30
   b. 60–80
   c. 40–60
   d. 20–40

4. Atrial activity is not discerned on an EKG strip in all of the following rhythms except:
   a. IVR
   b. AIVR
   c. A fib
   d. V tach

5. Ventricular diastole refers to ventricular:
   a. Contraction   c. Systole
   b. Relaxation   d. Pressure ratio

6. The heart ventricle with the thickest myocardium is the:
   a. Right   b. Left

7. The coronary arteries receive oxygenated blood from the: *from the ventricle*
   a. Aorta   c. Pulmonary veins
   b. Coronary sinus   d. Pulmonary arteries

8. The QRS interval should normally be
   _____ seconds or smaller.
   a. 0.20   c. 0.18
   b. 0.12   d. 0.36

9. Oscilloscopic evidence of ventricular fibrillation can be mimicked by artifact.
   a. True   b. False

10. The neurotransmitter for the parasympathetic nervous system is acetylcholine. Release of acetylcholine:
    1. Slows the heart rate
    2. Increases the heart rate
    3. Slows atrioventricular conduction
    4. Increases atrioventricular conduction
    a. 1 and 3
    b. 2 and 3
    c. 3 and 4
    d. 1 and 4

11. The most notable characteristic of asystole is the total absence of waveforms on an EKG strip or cardiac monitor.
    a. True   b. False

12. It may be difficult to distinguish asystole from very fine V fib; therefore, you must always check _____ different leads in order to definitively identify asystole.
    a. Four   c. Two
    b. Three   d. Five

13. PEA is not an actual rhythm; rather, it represents a clinical condition wherein the patient is clinically dead, despite the fact that some type of organized rhythm appears on the monitor.
    a. True   b. False

14. This rhythm resembles a turning about or twisting motion along the baseline (isoelectric line).
    a. Ventricular tachycardia
    b. Ventricular asystole
    c. Torsades de pointes
    d. Pulseless electrical activity

15. PEA, a life-threatening dysrhythmia, may result from:
    a. Hypokalemia
    b. Hypomagnesemia
    c. Tricyclic antidepressant drug overdose
    d. All the above

REVIEW STRIPS

1. Rate _____   Rhythm _____

   P wave _____   PR interval _____

   QRS complex _____   Interpretation _____

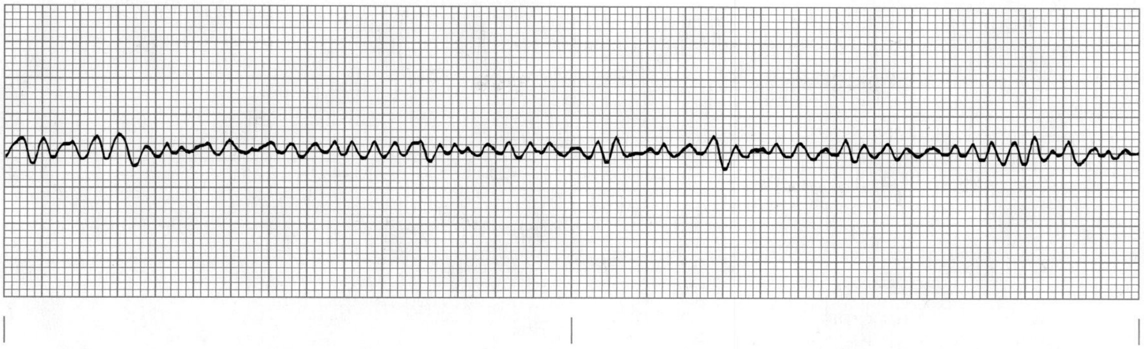

2. Rate _____   Rhythm _____

   P wave _____   PR interval _____

   QRS complex _____   Interpretation _____

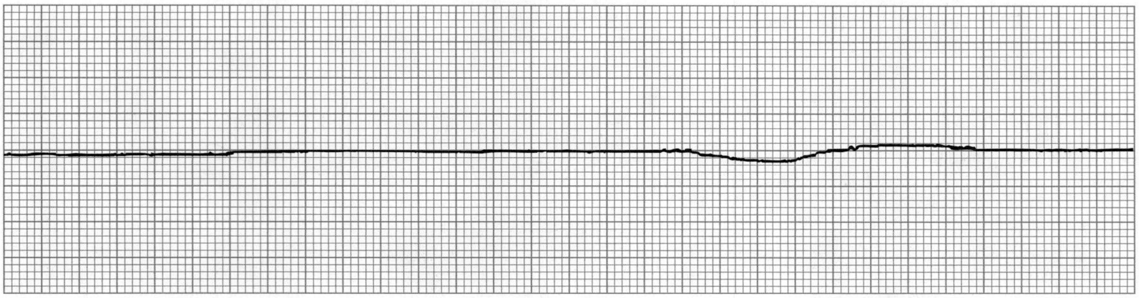

3. Rate _____   Rhythm _____

   P wave _____   PR interval _____

   QRS complex _____   Interpretation _____

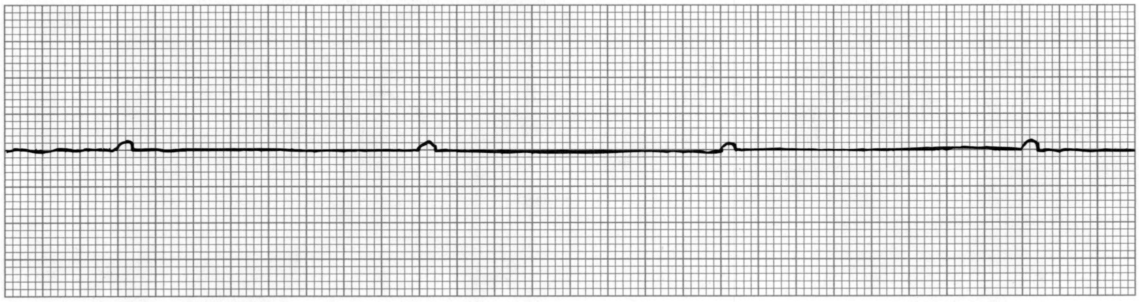

4. Rate _____   Rhythm _____

   P wave _____   PR interval _____

   QRS complex _____   Interpretation _____

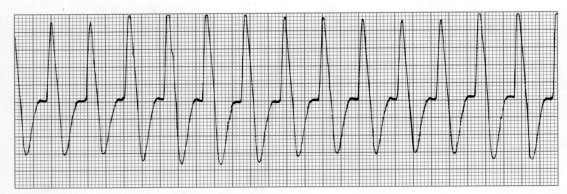

5. Rate _____   Rhythm _____

    P wave _____   PR interval _____

    QRS complex _____   Interpretation _____

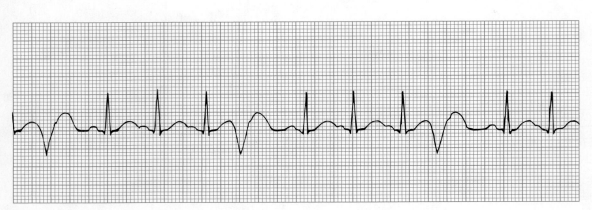

6. Rate _____   Rhythm _____

    P wave _____   PR interval _____

    QRS complex _____   Interpretation _____

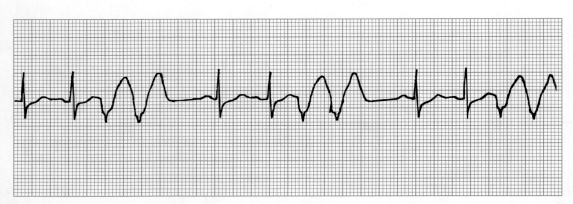

7. Rate _____   Rhythm _____

    P wave _____   PR interval _____

    QRS complex _____   Interpretation _____

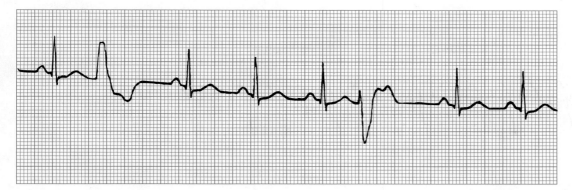

8. Rate _____   Rhythm _____

   P wave _____   PR interval _____

   QRS complex _____   Interpretation _____

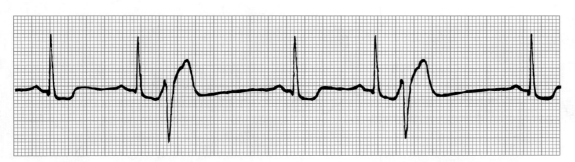

9. Rate _____   Rhythm _____

   P wave _____   PR interval _____

   QRS complex _____   Interpretation _____

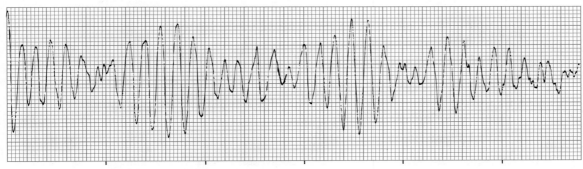

10. Rate _____   Rhythm _____

    P wave _____   PR interval _____

    QRS complex _____   Interpretation _____

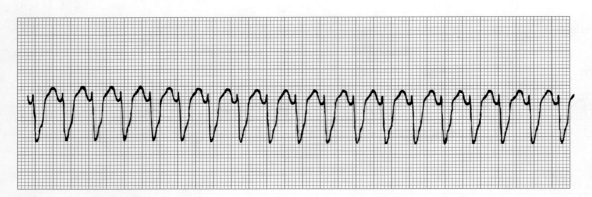

11. Rate _____   Rhythm _____

    P wave _____   PR interval _____

    QRS complex _____   Interpretation _____

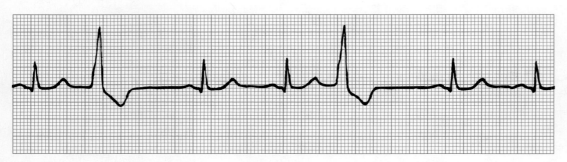

12. Rate _____   Rhythm _____

    P wave _____   PR interval _____

    QRS complex _____   Interpretation _____

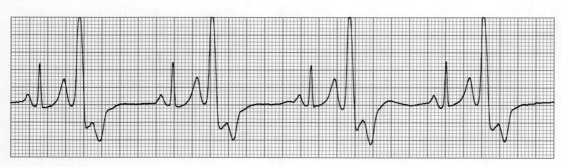

13. Rate _____   Rhythm _____

    P wave _____   PR interval _____

    QRS complex _____   Interpretation _____

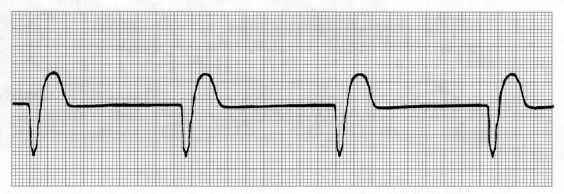

14. Rate _____   Rhythm _____

    P wave _____   PR interval _____

    QRS complex _____   Interpretation _____

Objectives

Upon completion of this chapter, the student will be able to:

■ Explain the electrical conduction system of the heart

■ Describe and identify first-degree atrioventricular block, including EKG characteristics

■ Discuss and identify second-degree atrioventricular block (Mobitz type I or Wenckebach), including EKG characteristics

■ Describe and identify second-degree atrioventricular block (Mobitz type II), including EKG characteristics

■ Explain and identify third-degree atrioventricular block (complete), including EKG characteristics

■ Discuss the clinical significance of the heart block rhythms

heart blocks electrical conduction system disorders

first-degree heart block the most usual form of block, results from excessive conduction delay in the AV node

Introducing the Heart Block Rhythms

INTRODUCTION

In this chapter we deal with rhythms that are primarily disorders of conduction. These rhythms occur when the electrical impulses that originate in the sinoatrial (SA) node are blocked or delayed in an area of the heart's electrical conduction system. You have already learned the importance of using the five-step approach to EKG interpretation in previous chapters, and this systematic approach is imperative in order for you to truly understand the heart blocks. Again, memorization is not acceptable—you must comprehend and commit to memory the characteristics of each heart block. If you focus on learning rather than memorizing these characteristics, you will gain a thorough and lasting understanding of the electrical conduction system disorders called **heart blocks**.

The discussion in this chapter classifies the heart blocks according to the degree of blockage. Heart blocks that are considered *partial,* or *incomplete,* include first-degree atrioventricular (AV) block, second-degree block (Mobitz type I or Wenckebach), and second-degree block (Mobitz type II). Third-degree heart block stands alone as the only *complete* heart block. Disorders of conduction may be either permanent or transient, minor or significant. As in all dysrhythmias, the seriousness of the heart blocks must be based on the patient's overall clinical appearance. 3/24/16

FIRST-DEGREE ATRIOVENTRICULAR BLOCK

First-degree heart block is the most usual form of block. Typically, first-degree block results from excessive conduction delay in the AV node. The impulse conduction between the atria and the bundle of His is delayed at the level of the AV node. Because of this delay, the PR interval (PRI, which would normally be less than 0.20 sec) will be prolonged.

First-degree heart block is the least serious type of heart blocks and is not actually a dysrhythmia. Its presence indicates only a delay at the AV node, rather than a definite block, and is sometimes called first-degree AV block. In fact, first-degree block is included in the description of the underlying rhythm and may be stated as "sinus bradycardia with first-degree block" or "sinus rhythm with first-degree block."

As you continue to learn to interpret EKG strips, you may tend to identify a first-degree block incorrectly if you do not carefully apply the five-step approach that you have learned in this text. At first glance, first-degree block may closely resemble normal sinus rhythm because all parameters are within normal limits *except for the PR interval*. But if you carefully apply *each* of the five steps, you will note that the PR interval is greater than *0.20* seconds and, therefore, the rhythm is not normal.

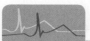 **TABLE 11–1 First-degree AV block**

Questions 1–5	Answers
1. What is the rate?	Based on the rate of the underlying rhythm
2. What is the rhythm?	Usually regular
3. Is there a P wave before each QRS?	Yes
Are the P waves upright and uniform?	Yes
4. What is the length of the PR interval?	Greater than 0.20 sec (3–5 small squares)
5. Do all the QRS complexes look alike?	Yes
What is the length of the QRS complexes?	Less than 0.12 sec (3 small squares)

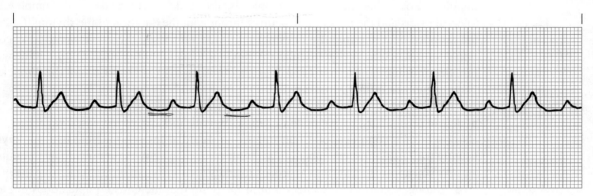

FIGURE 11–1. First-degree AV block

First-degree heart block may occur in patients who have no history of underlying heart disease, and it is sometimes seen in young athletes. This delay in conduction may also be seen in patients who are taking prescribed medications, such as beta-blockers, calcium channel blockers, and digoxin. If a patient has been diagnosed with an acute myocardial infarction, you must be particularly alert and carefully monitor and closely observe the patient for the development of more serious heart blocks.

Now it's time to analyze an EKG strip by applying the five-step approach in order to prove that all components of the five-step approach are indeed normal, with the exception of the PR interval. (See ■ **Table 11–1** and ■ **Figure 11–1**.)

In Figure 11–1, you should note the heart rate as 70 beats per minute (BPM), the rhythm is regular, P waves are present and upright, the PRI is 0.24 seconds, and the QRS is 0.04 seconds. These findings should validate First-Degree Heart Block.

Remember that a prolonged PR interval is the hallmark of first-degree block and is most commonly the only variation in the EKG strip. Also remember that first-degree block looks very much like normal sinus rhythm, but the PR interval is greater than 0.20 seconds. **Remember . . . always monitor your patient's clinical condition!**

SECOND-DEGREE HEART BLOCKS

Now we will discuss the two types of *second-degree heart block*. Atrioventricular (AV) block can be defined as a delay or interruption in the transmission of an impulse, either transient or permanent, from the atria to the ventricles. This delay may be due to an anatomic or functional impairment in the conduction system. The conduction can be delayed, intermittent, or absent. The first type of the second-degree blocks is less serious than the second type because bradycardia is less likely to be present and because cardiac output is less likely to be seriously decreased in a second-degree type I block.

The variety of names assigned to the two types of second-degree blocks are those of the two physicians who initially identified and described these heart blocks: Karel F. Wenckebach (1864–1940), a Dutch-Austrian physician, and Woldemar Mobitz (1889–1951), a German physician. Both were instrumental in the research, classification, and investigation of these two types of heart blocks.

Second-degree atrioventricular block (Mobitz type I or Wenckebach)

second-degree AV block, Mobitz type I, or Wenckebach progressive prolongation of the electrical impulse delay at the AV node, which produces an increase in the length of the PR interval

The progressive prolongation of the electrical impulse delay at the AV node produces an increase in the length of the PR interval in **second-degree AV block**. A characteristic cyclic pattern is produced: The PR interval continues to increase in length until such time as the impulse is not conducted or a QRS complex is "dropped." After the "dropped" complex, the PR interval resets and the pattern is repetitive throughout the duration of the rhythm. Because of the dropped beat, the impulse does not reach the ventricles; therefore, ventricular contraction does not occur. The ventricular rhythm is irregular, but the atrial rhythm remains regular. Second-degree Mobitz type I heart block is also referred to as the Wenckebach phenomenon or simply Mobitz type I.

Mobitz I may be caused by abnormal conduction of the electrical impulses at the AV node and precipitated by AV node ischemia, digitalis therapy, or increased vagal tone. It may also occur as a complication of an inferior myocardial infarction. Note that this rhythm is usually transient, most often benign and will often resolve without outside intervention.

As you apply the five-step approach to analyze this rhythm, you should note the progressive prolongation of the PR interval until the point that the QRS complex does not appear. (See ■ **Table 11–2** and ■ **Figures 11–2a, 11–2b, 11–2c**.)

In Figure 11–2a, you should note the heart rate as 60 BPM, the rhythm is irregular, P waves are present and upright, the PRI progressively prolongs until a QRS complex is dropped, and the QRS is 0.04 seconds. These findings should validate Second-Degree Heart Block, Mobitz I.

In Figure 11–2b, you should note the heart rate as 70 BPM, the rhythm is irregular, P waves are present and upright, the PRI progressively prolongs until a QRS complex is dropped, and the QRS is 0.06 seconds. These findings should validate Second-Degree Heart Block, Mobitz I.

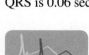

TABLE 11–2 Second-degree block, Mobitz type I

Questions 1–5	Answers
1. What is the rate?	Atrial unaffected; ventricular rate is usually slower than atrial
2. What is the rhythm?	Atrial rhythm regular; ventricular rhythm irregular
3. Is there a P wave before each QRS?	Yes
Are the P waves upright and uniform?	Yes, for conducted beats
4. What is the length of the PR interval?	Progressively prolongs until a QRS is not conducted
5. Do all the QRS complexes look alike?	Yes
What is the length of the QRS complexes?	Less than 0.12 sec

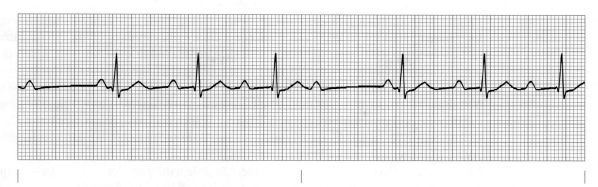

FIGURE 11–2a. Second-degree heart block, Mobitz type I, Wenckebach

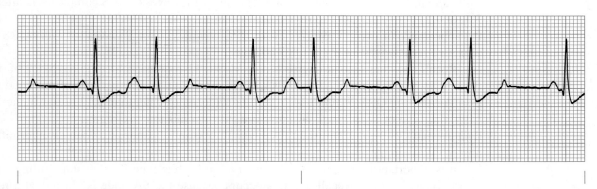

FIGURE 11–2b. Second-degree heart block, Mobitz type I, Wenckebach

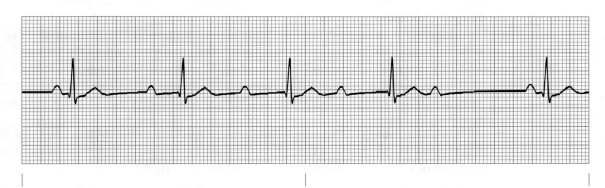

FIGURE 11–2c. Second-degree heart block, Mobitz type I, Wenckebach

In Figure 11–2c, you should note the heart rate as 50 BPM, the rhythm is irregular, P waves are present and upright, the PRI progressively prolongs until a QRS complex is dropped, and the QRS is 0.04 seconds. These findings should validate Sinus Bradycardia with Second-Degree Heart Block, Mobitz I.

Remember that a progressively prolonging PR interval is the *key* to recognizing second-degree Mobitz I heart block. **Remember . . . always monitor your patient's clinical condition!**

3/24/16

Second-degree atrioventricular block (Mobitz type II)

Second-degree AV block, or Mobitz type II, is a more serious dysrhythmia than either first-degree block or Mobitz type I. This is because type II indicates an increased risk of

second-degree AV block, or Mobitz type II a more serious dysrhythmia that occurs when there is an intermittent interruption in the electrical conduction system near or below the AV junction

progression to third-degree, or complete, heart block. Mobitz type II occurs when there is an intermittent interruption in the electrical conduction system near or below the AV junction.

To understand this dysrhythmia, you should understand that the SA node is functionally unimpaired. In other words, the SA node is generating electrical impulses at regular intervals. Therefore, you should note that P waves will occur in a regular pattern across the EKG strip. You should also note, however, that some P waves are not followed by a QRS complex, because the impulse is completely blocked in one bundle branch and periodically blocked in the other bundle branch (these blocks are referred to as *bundle branch blocks*). We earlier referred to the AV node as the "gatekeeper" to the ventricles, so it may be helpful to remember now that in Mobitz type II, the gate closes at regular intervals. When the gate closes, the impulse cannot be conducted through the bundle of His to the ventricles; thus no QRS complex is produced.

Second-degree blocks are often referred to by the ratio of P waves to QRS complexes. This ratio may vary or may be constant. The ratio of P waves to QRS complexes is often 2:1, 3:1, or 4:1. It may be easier to remember that an EKG strip of Mobitz type II may present as the appearance of two P waves for every QRS complex, three P waves for every QRS complex, or four P waves for every QRS complex.

Recall now that second-degree block, Mobitz II, represents a complete block of one of the bundle branches and a partial block of the other branch. It is because of this conduction disorder that the QRS complex will often be widened (greater than 0.12 sec). Characteristically, this type of heart block will produce PR intervals that are regular in length (for conducted beats), more P waves than QRS complexes, and a pattern that depicts intermittently absent QRS complexes.

It is important to note that the PR interval in Mobitz type II is constant, or regular, for every conducted beat. Recall that this occurs because the SA node is "firing" at a regular pace, but the impulse is blocked or is not allowed to be conducted at certain intervals. Whereas the atrial rhythm is regular, the ventricular rhythm is irregular because of the dropped or nonconducted beats.

Mobitz II may be associated with septal wall necrosis, acute myocardial infarction, acute myocarditis, or advanced coronary artery disease. Depending on the ventricular rate, the patient may be symptomatic or asymptomatic. If the ventricular rate is fast enough to sustain cardiac output at an effective level, the patient may not exhibit overt signs or symptoms. In this heart block, it is more common for the patient to exhibit signs or symptoms of decreased perfusion.

Review ■ **Table 11–3** and apply the five-step approach to the rhythm strips that follow in ■ **Figures 11–3a, 11–3b, 11–3c.** As you review the table and strip illustrations, consider the effect of a 2:1 block on cardiac output and overall perfusion.

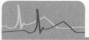

TABLE 11–3 Second-degree block, Mobitz II

Questions 1–5	Answers
1. What is the rate?	Atrial rate regular; ventricular rate may be bradycardic
2. What is the rhythm?	Atrial rhythm regular; ventricular rhythm irregular
3. Is there a P wave before each QRS? Are the P waves upright and uniform?	Yes; some P waves are not followed by a QRS complex P waves are usually upright and uniform
4. What is the length of the PR interval?	Constant for conducted beats
5. Do all the QRS complexes look alike? What is the length of the QRS complexes?	Yes; intermittently absent Less than or greater than 0.12 sec

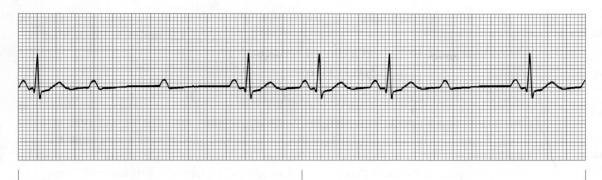

FIGURE 11–3a. Second-degree heart block, Mobitz type II

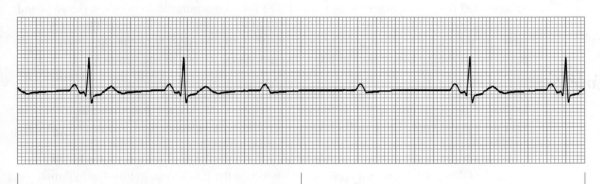

FIGURE 11–3b. Second-degree heart block, Mobitz type II

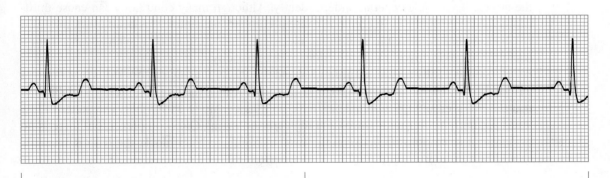

FIGURE 11–3c. Second-degree heart block, Mobitz type II

In Figure 11–3a, you should note the heart rate as 50 BPM, the atrial rhythm is regular, ventricular rhythm is irregular, P waves are present and upright, the PRI interval is 0.18 seconds and constant (regular) for conducted beats, and the QRS is 0.04 seconds. These findings should validate Second-Degree Heart Block, Mobitz II.

In Figure 11–3b, you should note the heart rate as 40 BPM, the atrial rhythm is regular, ventricular rhythm is irregular, P waves are present and upright, the PRI interval is 0.16 seconds and constant (regular) for conducted beats, and the QRS is 0.04 seconds. These findings should validate Second-Degree Heart Block, Mobitz II.

In Figure 11–3c, you should note the heart rate as 60 BPM, the atrial rhythm is regular and the ventricular rhythm is regular, P waves are present and upright, the PRI interval is 0.16 seconds and constant (regular) for conducted beats, and the QRS is 0.06 seconds. These findings should validate Sinus Bradycardia with Second-Degree Heart Block, Mobitz II, 2:1.

third-degree AV block (complete) the most serious type of heart block; the atria and ventricles are completely blocked or separated from each other electrically at or below the AV node; ventricular rate will most commonly be between 20 and 40 BPM

Pacemaker from bundle of his or purkini fibers.

Remember that the keys to interpreting Mobitz Type II include the constancy of the PR intervals (for conducted beats) and intermittently <u>absent QRS complexes</u>. **Remember . . . always monitor your patient's clinical condition!**

3/24/16

THIRD-DEGREE ATRIOVENTRICULAR BLOCK (COMPLETE)

Third-degree AV block (complete) is, without question, the most serious type of heart block. This is true because third-degree block may progress to asystole and because the ventricular rate is usually very <u>slow and ineffective</u>. The heart rate of the ventricles may not be able to maintain a sufficient cardiac output needed to sustain life. Consequently, complete heart block (CHB) is referred to as a lethal dysrhythmia.

In the truest sense of the term *complete,* the atria and ventricles are completely blocked or separated from each other electrically. There is no communication between the atria and ventricles, as they literally beat independently of each other. The SA node fires at regular intervals, producing P waves at its normal rate of <u>60</u> to <u>100 BPM</u>, whereas the ventricles are paced by an escape pacemaker in either the junctional tissues or the ventricles. If the ventricular pacemaker is the escape pacemaker, the ventricular rate will most commonly be between <u>20</u> and <u>40 BPM</u>. If the resulting QRS complex is narrow, the escape pacemaker is located in the junctional tissue. If the QRS is widened, the escape pacemaker is located in the Purkinje network. There is, therefore, no relationship between the P waves and the QRS complexes.

The PR intervals will be variable in length. Some P waves may actually be "buried" inside the QRS complex and, therefore, not visible on the EKG strip. In this dysrhythmia, the gate actually closes and does not permit conduction of the initial electrical impulse through the AV junction or ventricles. This dysrhythmia is sometimes called AV dissociation because the atria and ventricles operate independently. Although many conditions can cause third-degree heart block, the most common cause is coronary ischemia. This heart block may also result from degenerative changes in the electrical conduction system (with advanced age), acute myocarditis, myocardial infarction, or drug toxicity.

As you carefully review ■ **Table 11–4** and the accompanying rhythm strips in ■ **Figures 11–4a, 11–4b, 11–4c** you will recognize that the PR intervals are completely variable and that the P waves and QRS complexes have no relationship to each other. The pattern illustrates regularly occurring P waves and regularly occurring QRS complexes, but there is no evidence of a relationship between the two. In complete heart block, the R-to-R intervals should be constant.

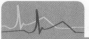

TABLE 11–4 Third-degree (complete) heart block

Questions 1–5	Answers
1. What is the rate?	Atrial rate usually 60–100 BPM; ventricular rate based on site of escape pacemaker
2. What is the rhythm?	Atrial rhythm regular; ventricular rhythm regular
3. Is there a P wave before each QRS? Are the P waves upright and uniform?	No relationship to QRS complexes Yes
4. What is the length of the PR interval?	Totally variable; no pattern
5. Do all the QRS complexes look alike? What is the length of the QRS complexes?	Yes Based on site of escape pacemaker

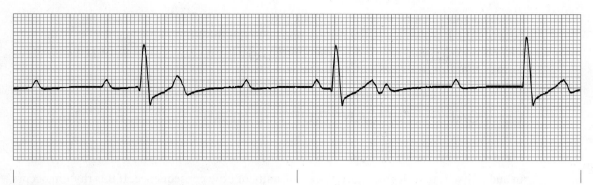

FIGURE 11–4a. Third-degree heart block

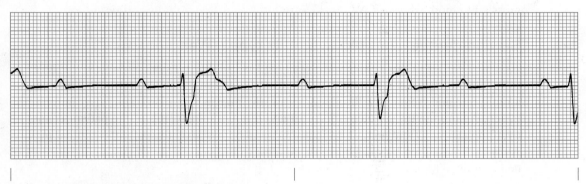

FIGURE 11–4b. Third-degree heart block

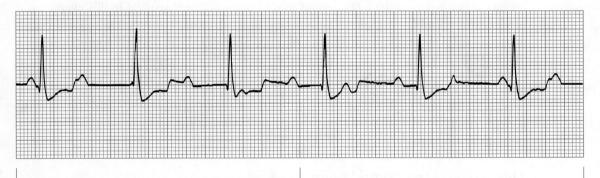

FIGURE 11–4c. Third-degree heart block

In Figure 11–4a, you should note the heart rate as 30 BPM, the atrial rhythm is regular and the ventricular rhythm is regular, P waves are present and upright with no relationship to the QRS complexes, the PRI is variable with no pattern, and the QRS is 0.10 seconds. These findings should validate Third-Degree Heart Block.

In Figure 11–4b, you should note the heart rate as 20 BPM, the atrial rhythm is regular and the ventricular rhythm is regular, P waves are present and upright with no relationship to the QRS complexes, the PRI is variable with no pattern, and the QRS is greater than 0.12 seconds. These findings should validate Third-Degree Heart Block.

In Figure 11–4c, you should note the heart rate as 60 BPM, the atrial rhythm is regular and the ventricular rhythm is regular, P waves are present and upright with no relationship to the QRS complexes, the PRI is variable with no pattern, and the QRS is 0.08 seconds. These findings should validate Third-Degree Heart Block.

Remember that complete heart block produces an EKG strip that shows no relationship between the P waves and QRS complexes; however, the atrial rate is regular, as is the ventricular rate. It is imperative that you observe the patient closely. **You must remember . . . always monitor your patient's clinical condition!**

CLINICAL SIGNIFICANCE OF THE HEART BLOCK RHYTHMS

First-degree heart block

In and of itself, first-degree heart block is usually of little consequence. If this rhythm occurs in the face of an acute myocardial infarction, the patient must be closely observed and frequently assessed. Keep in mind, however, that this dysrhythmia may signal an initial progression to more advanced AV block.

Second-degree heart block, Mobitz type I (Wenckebach)

As stated earlier in this chapter, Mobitz type I is usually transient and often will revert to the patient's normal rhythm without outside intervention. If the EKG pattern demonstrates a rapid rate and frequently "dropped" beats, the patient's cardiac output may be compromised. Again, the importance of careful and diligent monitoring of the patient cannot be overemphasized. Treatment, if indicated, should be based on the patient's clinical picture. As with first-degree block, you must be alert to the possibility of advancing degrees of heart block.

Second-degree heart block, Mobitz type II

Mobitz II is the first of the more serious blocks that we have discussed in this chapter. It is prudent to remember that, often, Mobitz type II heart block will progress to third-degree heart block. Furthermore, the frequency of dropped beats (absences of QRS complexes) is a major concern in monitoring a patient who presents with this rhythm.

Recall that cardiac output may be seriously compromised. Be alert for signs and symptoms of decreased perfusion. These signs and symptoms may include syncope, dizziness, decreased level of consciousness, angina, and other indications of hypoperfusion. If the patient presents with symptoms, you should consider and follow local protocols for treatment, as appropriate.

Third-degree (complete) heart block

Recall now that third-degree heart block is generally considered a lethal dysrhythmia, and act accordingly! The signs and symptoms exhibited by the patient who presents with third-degree block may be indicative of severe hypoperfusion; however, it is important to note that this is not *always* the case. Pay close attention to the width of the QRS complexes in order to determine whether the pacemaker site is ventricular or junctional.

By way of review, you should remember that the heart rate is based on the site of the pacemaker. If the QRS complexes are narrow and the patient is asymptomatic, the pacemaker cells in the AV junctional tissue are most likely serving as the pacemaker site. In this case the symptomatic patient may be treated with atropine, or pacing may be indicated. On the other hand, if the patient is exhibiting signs and symptoms and the QRS complexes are wide, transcutaneous pacing followed by the insertion of a transvenous pacemaker may be indicated.

Again, **listen to and observe** your patient, and never base your treatment decision on EKG strip analysis alone.

CHAPTER 11

 SUMMARY

Rhythms that are primarily disorders of conduction are called heart blocks. These rhythms occur when the electrical impulses that originate in the SA node are blocked or delayed in an area of the heart's electrical conduction system. Careful attention to, and evaluation of, the PR intervals is a critical component in the proper analysis of heart block rhythms.

 KEY POINTS TO REMEMBER

1. In the vast majority of cases, heart blocks represent a conduction disorder.

2. The presence of a first-degree heart block indicates only a delay at the AV node rather than a definite block.

3. In second-degree AV block, Mobitz type I, the PR interval continues to increase in length until such time as the impulse is not conducted or a QRS complex is dropped.

4. Mobitz type I is also known as Wenckebach.

5. Second-degree AV block, Mobitz type II will produce PR intervals that are constant in length (for conducted beats).

6. In Mobitz type II, there are more P waves than QRS complexes, with a pattern that depicts intermittently absent QRS complexes.

7. Third-degree heart block is a *complete* heart block.

8. The atria and ventricles are completely blocked or separated from each other electrically in third-degree block.

9. In third-degree block, there is no communication between the atria and ventricles because they literally beat independently of each other.

10. In dealing with patients who present with a heart block, it is vitally important that a thorough patient assessment be conducted in order to determine the specific clinical significance of the block in that patient.

 REVIEW QUESTIONS

1. When the EKG shows there is no relationship between the P wave and the QRS complex, you should suspect:
   a. First-degree block
   b. Second-degree block
   c. Third-degree block
   d. Electromechanical dissociation

2. Wenckebach differs from complete heart block in that CHB usually has a:
   a. Faster rate
   b. Normal QRS
   c. Constant PR interval
   d. Regular RR interval

3. PAT is a sudden onset of atrial tachycardia.
   a. True
   b. False

4. The keys to interpretation of second-degree heart block, Mobitz type II, are the presence of constant PR intervals and the fact that there are more P waves present than QRS complexes.
   a. True
   b. False

5. In order to calculate heart rate accurately by the R-to-R interval method, the patient must have a regular rhythm.
   a. True
   b. False

6. Proper application of EKG chest electrodes includes all of the following except:
   a. Cleaning the patient's skin
   b. Drying the patient's skin
   c. Shaving the chest area of excess hair
   d. Cleaning each electrode prior to application

7. It is prudent to remember that, often, Mobitz type II heart block will progress to third-degree heart block.
   a. True   b. False

8. Typically, first-degree block results from excessive conduction delay in the:
   a. SA node   c. Internodal pathways
   b. AV node   d. Purkinje network

9. Lead II is the lead most commonly used in the pre-hospital arena because it:
   a. Is easier to apply
   b. Shows good T waves
   c. Illustrates good P waves
   d. Is faster to apply

10. The heart block rhythm that most closely resembles a normal sinus rhythm is:
    a. Third-degree heart block
    b. Second-degree, Mobitz type I
    c. First-degree heart block
    d. Atrioventricular dissociation

11. It is important to note that the PR interval in Mobitz type II is constant, or regular, for every conducted beat.
    a. True   b. False

12. The T wave on the EKG strip represents:
    a. Rest period
    b. Bundle of His
    c. Atrial contraction
    d. Ventricular contraction *or repolerization*

13. If the ventricular pacemaker is the escape pacemaker, the ventricular rate will most commonly be between 20 and 40 BPM.
    a. True   b. False

14. A constant and prolonged PR interval is the hallmark of _____ degree block and is most commonly the only variation in the EKG strip.
    a. First-   c. Second-, type I
    b. Third-   d. Second-, type II

15. The first type of second-degree block is more serious than the second type because bradycardia is less likely to be present and because cardiac output is less likely to be seriously decreased in a second-degree type I block.
    a. True   b. False

REVIEW STRIPS

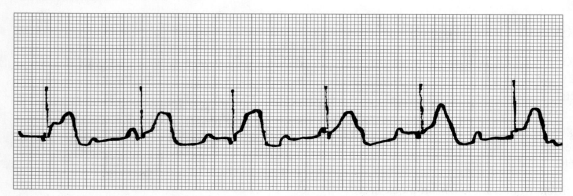

1. Rate _____   Rhythm _____

   P wave _____   PR interval _____

   QRS complex _____   Interpretation _____

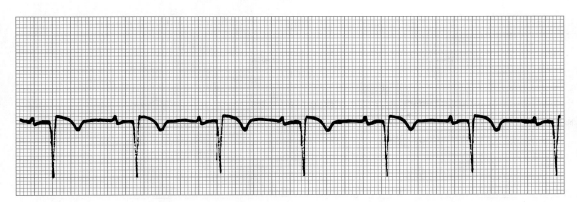

2. Rate _____   Rhythm _____

   P wave _____   PR interval _____

   QRS complex _____   Interpretation _____

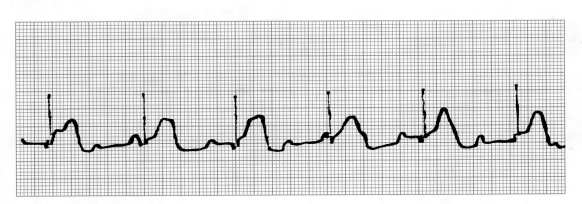

3. Rate _____   Rhythm _____

   P wave _____   PR interval _____

   QRS complex _____   Interpretation _____

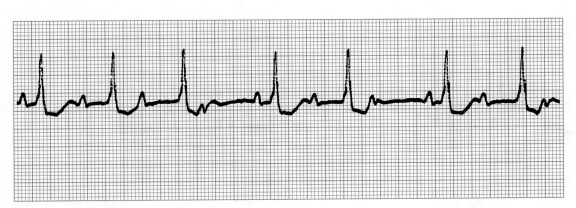

4. Rate _____   Rhythm _____

   P wave _____   PR interval _____

   QRS complex _____   Interpretation _____

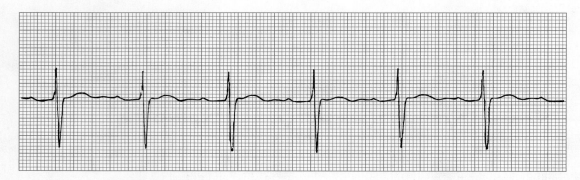

5. Rate _____   Rhythm _____

   P wave _____   PR interval _____

   QRS complex _____   Interpretation _____

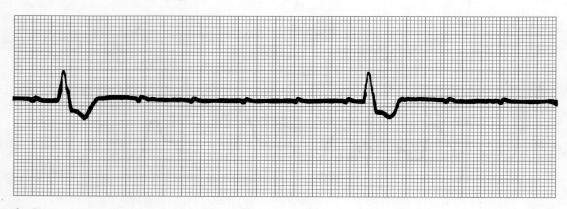

6. Rate _____   Rhythm _____

   P wave _____   PR interval _____

   QRS complex _____   Interpretation _____

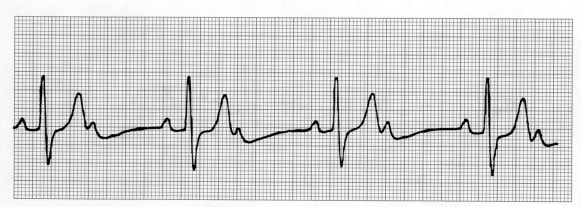

7. Rate _____   Rhythm _____

   P wave _____   PR interval _____

   QRS complex _____   Interpretation _____

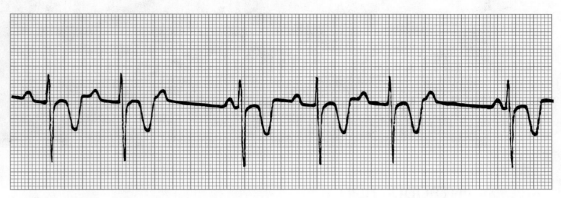

8. Rate _____   Rhythm _____

    P wave _____   PR interval _____

    QRS complex _____   Interpretation _____

Introducing the Pacemaker Rhythms

Objectives

Upon completion of this chapter, the student will be able to:

- Explain the concept of an artificial pacemaker
- Describe transcutaneous pacing
- Discuss transvenous pacing
- List three types of permanent pacemakers
- Identify the indications for pacing
- Discuss the rules for interpretation of the pacemaker rhythms
- List common problems associated with pacemakers
- Explain the clinical significance of pacemaker rhythms

artificial pacemaker a device that substitutes for the normal pacemaker cells of the heart's electrical conduction system

pacemaker spike EKG wave produced by an artificial pacemaker

generator controls the rate and strength of each electrical impulse

lead wires relay the electrical impulse from the generator to the myocardium

temporary pacemakers used to sustain a patient's heart rate in emergent situations

permanent pacemakers implanted inside the patient's upper left chest (most commonly) and are left in place

transcutaneous pacing (TCP) commonly called external cardiac pacing, consists of two large electrode pads, which are most commonly placed in an anterior-posterior position on the patient's chest to conduct electrical impulses through the skin to the heart

INTRODUCTION

An **artificial pacemaker** can be thought of as a medical device that substitutes for the normal pacemaker cells of the heart's electrical conduction system by the use of electrical impulses. An artificial pacemaker is, in the truest sense of the concept, an artificial regulator of heart rate. The use of artificial pacemakers may be necessitated when a patient's inherent electrical conduction pathway fails to function sufficiently. The EKG wave produced by an artificial pacemaker is referred to as a **pacemaker spike**.

Patients who experience signs and symptoms related to extensive disease of the sinus node (sick sinus syndrome), symptomatic bradycardia, or symptomatic complete heart block are often prime candidates for artificial pacing. Artificial pacemaker technology is advancing rapidly and is complex in nature. In this chapter, we will discuss some basic concepts regarding artificial pacemakers and the rhythms they produce. It is important for the health care professional to be able to recognize the presence of pacemaker rhythms on EKG strips in order to make prudent decisions about treatment.

Whether temporary or permanent, artificial pacemakers are small devices that initiate electrical impulses in specific locations in the myocardial tissue. Artificial pacemakers have two basic parts: the generator and the lead wires. The **generator** controls the rate and strength of each electrical impulse. The **lead wires** have an electrode at the tip and relay the electrical impulse from the generator to the myocardium.

Temporary pacemakers are used to sustain a patient's heart rate in emergent situations, whereas **permanent pacemakers** are implanted inside the patient's upper left chest (most commonly) and are left in place. The following discussion provides an overview of common considerations regarding artificial pacemakers.

TEMPORARY PACING

Transcutaneous pacing

Transcutaneous pacing, often abbreviated **TCP**, is also commonly called external cardiac pacing. Initially introduced in the early 1950s, TCP was used to treat serious symptoms associated with complete heart block. The device quickly fell out of favor, primarily because of its marked disadvantages, such as patients' complaints of associated pain and EKG aberrations secondary to muscle contractions. Only in the past 20 years have modern technological advances made TCP an acceptable and often effective modality for rhythms such as symptomatic bradycardia, symptomatic complete heart block, and other rhythm disturbances.

The American Heart Association (AHA) has now recognized and recommended the use of TCP devices in the bradycardia algorithm. Because TCP can be initiated quickly and is not as invasive as other pacing methods, the AHA has recommended it as the suggested treatment of choice in emergent cardiac care settings.

Transcutaneous pacing consists of two large electrode pads, which are most commonly placed in an anterior-posterior position on the patient's chest to conduct electrical impulses through the skin to the heart. Utilizing this method, the cardiac muscle cells depolarize in a normal fashion.

Before the implementation of TCP, the patient should be placed in a supine position, and an IV/IO, oxygen, and EKG monitoring must be established. Most prehospital care systems require that the prehospital provider receive orders from medical control prior to initiating TCP; however, others may operate with standing orders in place.

Symptomatic bradycardia must be confirmed prior to implementing TCP procedures. After the electrode pads and the electrodes are properly placed the desired heart rate should be set. Unlike manual defibrillation, the three lead and four lead cable electrodes must be in place, as well as pacer pads, in order for pacing to work. This rate is commonly in the range of 60 to 80 beats per minute (BPM). The initial voltage setting is at 0 milliamperes (mA) before the pacer is turned on.

Although recommendations vary regarding initial current settings, it is universally agreed that the ampere setting be *gradually* increased until capture is accomplished. **Capture** is usually noted by the presence of a spike and wide QRS complexes, the presence of an adequate carotid pulse and blood pressure, and an increased level of consciousness. The prehospital provider must be in voice contact with medical control, and the patient's overall clinical condition must be constantly monitored. Keep in mind that the preset heart rate and the amperage may need to be adjusted because of various factors, such as the patient's movement or changes in the patient's underlying heart rhythm. Rhythm strips should be gathered, and concise, detailed documentation is required. At times, the patient may experience pain and mild discomfort secondary to TCP implementation; therefore, sedation should be considered. In many areas of the country, the medical control must be contacted for sedation orders; however, you are advised to follow your local protocols.

Transvenous pacing

Transvenous (through a vein) pacing is another method for delivering electrical impulses to the myocardial tissue and is commonly held to be more reliable than transcutaneous pacing. In **transvenous pacing**, a lead wire is inserted through the skin, threaded into a large vein leading into the right side of the heart, and controlled by an external power source. The electrical impulses generated by the external power source stimulate the right atrium or the right ventricle and travel through the electrical conduction system, producing depolarization. Note that transvenous pacing is more invasive in nature than TCP, due to the necessity of venipuncture for the purpose of inserting the lead wire.

Pacemakers are preset, or programmed, to pace (or deliver electrical impulses) in two modes. A **fixed-rate, or asynchronous, pacemaker** is programmed to deliver electrical impulses at a constant selected rate. A **demand, or synchronous, pacemaker** generates electrical impulses when the patient's heart rate falls below a predetermined rate. Fixed-rate pacemakers are not commonly used in today's advanced technology.

PERMANENT PACING

Permanent, or implanted, pacemakers are most commonly used when patients present with signs of symptomatic bradycardia or complete heart block that have not responded to pharmacologic interventions. As stated earlier in this chapter, a permanent pacemaker consists of

capture noted by the presence of a spike and wide QRS complexes, the presence of an adequate carotid pulse and blood pressure, and an increased level of consciousness

transvenous pacing (through a vein) a lead wire is inserted through the skin and threaded into a large vein leading into the right side of the heart and controlled by an external power source

fixed-rate, or asynchronous, pacemaker programmed to deliver electrical impulses at a constant selected rate

demand, or synchronous, pacemaker generates electrical impulses when the patient's heart rate falls below a predetermined rate

a surgically implanted generator and a lead wire that is introduced into the heart through a central vein.

The three primary types of permanent pacemakers used today are the atrial, ventricular, and atrioventricular (AV) sequential pacemakers. Descriptions of these three types follow:

a. **Atrial pacemakers**—Atrial pacemakers are also known as single-chamber pacemakers. The lead wire electrode is inserted into the right atrium. The pacemaker's electrical impulse first stimulates the atrium and then travels down the electrical conduction pathway through the ventricles. (See ■ **Figure 12–1**.)

b. **Ventricular pacemakers**—Ventricular pacemakers are also known as single-chamber pacemakers. The lead wire electrode is inserted into the right ventricle. The electrical impulse from the pacemaker generator produces ventricular depolarization. (See ■ **Figure 12–2**.)

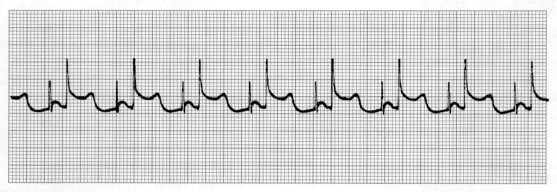

FIGURE 12–1. Atrial pacemaker

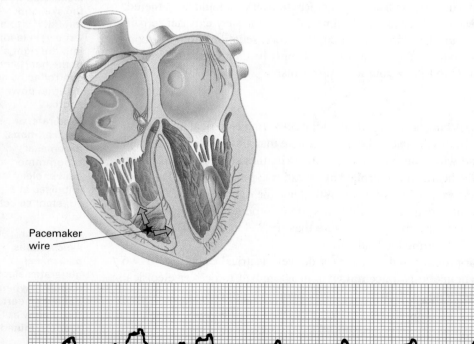

Pacemaker wire

FIGURE 12–2. Ventricular pacemaker

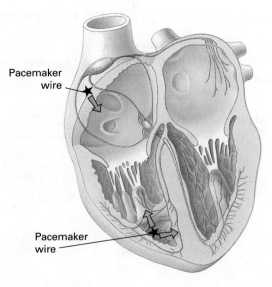

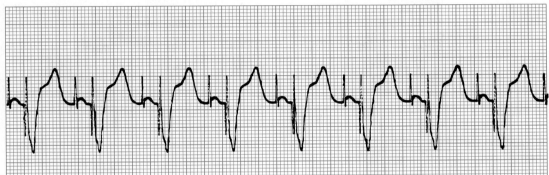

FIGURE 12–3. Atrioventricular sequential pacemaker

    c. AV sequential pacemakers—AV sequential pacemakers are also known as dual-chamber pacemakers. This is the most commonly used type of permanent pacemaker. There are two electrodes on the lead wire: One is placed in the right atrium and one is placed in the right ventricle. Artificial impulses stimulate, or pace, first the atria, then the ventricles. (See ■ **Figure 12–3.**)

New generation demand pacers may also have incorporated in their design, an implantable cardioverter defibrillator (ICD) designed to directly treat a cardiac tachydysrhythmia. Pacers that are older than 10 years may lack this capability. ICDs are often implanted in patients who are thought to be at high risk of sudden cardiac death, often due to ventricular tachycardia or ventricular fibrillation. ICDs may be described as implantable devices capable of delivering enough energy to defibrillate the heart without the need for a lead in or on the heart.

INDICATIONS FOR PACING

Artificial pacemakers may be indicated for patients who present with persistent and symptomatic second-degree type II heart block, complete heart block, occurrences of severe symptomatic bradycardia, or sick sinus syndrome. Transcutaneous pacing may be used as a temporary bridge modality in severe, symptomatic bradycardia-related rhythms, until transvenous pacing or permanent pacing can be established. Transcutaneous pacing may also be used in profound bradycardia, secondary to drug overdose, or in the rare event of failure of a permanent pacemaker.

RULES FOR INTERPRETATION OF PACEMAKER RHYTHMS

While analyzing an EKG strip produced by an artificial pacemaker, you should apply the five-step approach, just as you have done with the dysrhythmias in the previous chapters of this text. Consider ■ **Table 12–1** and ■ **Figure 12–4**.

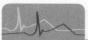 **TABLE 12–1 Artificial pacemaker rhythm**

Questions 1–5	Answers
1. What is the rate?	Varies according to preset rate of pacemaker
2. What is the rhythm?	Regular if pacing is fixed; irregular if demand-paced
3. Is there a P wave before each QRS?	May be absent or present, depending on type of artificial pacemaker
Are the P waves upright and uniform?	Pacemaker rhythm
4. What is the length of the PR interval?	Variable, depending on type of artificial pacemaker
5. Do all the QRS complexes look alike?	Usually; bizarre morphology; presence of spikes
What is the length of the QRS complexes?	Greater than 0.12 sec

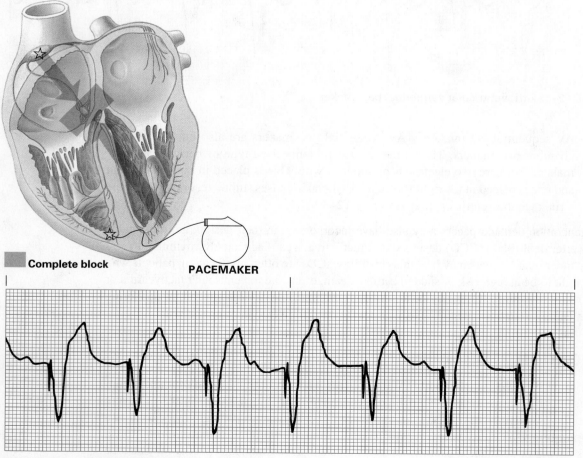

Complete block

PACEMAKER

FIGURE 12–4. Artificial pacemaker rhythm

In Figure 12–4, you should note the heart rate as 70 BPM, the rhythm is regular, P waves are not present, no PRI is discernible and the QRS is 0.12 seconds and has a pacer spike before the complex. These findings should validate Artificial Ventricular Pacer.

Remember that properly functioning pacemakers will produce rhythms with pacemaker spikes. The pacemaker spikes are usually readily identifiable; however, many of the newer cardiac monitors denote the pacemaker spike on either the oscilloscope or the graph paper or print an arrow at the bottom of the complex. It is essential that you realize that the presence of pacemaker spikes indicates only that the pacemaker is firing; pacemaker spikes do not reveal information relative to ventricular contraction. Assess your patient for the presence of symptoms. **Remember . . . always monitor your patient's clinical condition!**

COMMON PROBLEMS ASSOCIATED WITH PACEMAKERS

Battery failure

Decreased amplitude of the pacemaker spike and a slowing pacemaker rate may both be caused by battery failure. Most pacemaker batteries are based on today's modern technology and have long lives. Periodic pacemaker battery checks are usually made by the patient's physician, preventing the occurrence of battery failure. In the unlikely event of complete battery failure, the pacemaker will fail to function and the patient's underlying rhythm may return or cardiac arrest may result. Depending on the underlying rhythm and patient's symptoms, battery failure can be considered a dire emergency.

Runaway pacemakers

Fortunately, situations in which a pacemaker rhythm "runs away" are rarely seen today, especially with newer pacemakers. However, when this problem is identified, a rapid rate of electrical impulse discharge results. At times, the discharge rate may reach 200 to 300 BPM. Today's newer generators provide a gradual increase in rate as their battery currents decrease. Management of patients who exhibit evidence of runaway pacemaker rhythms consists of immediate transport to a definitive care facility.

Failure to capture

When an artificial pacemaker successfully depolarizes the specified chamber or chambers of the heart, as denoted by the presence of a pacemaker spike followed by a P wave or QRS complex, capture has occurred.

When lead wires become displaced or a pacemaker battery fails, the pacemaker can fail to capture. When failure to capture occurs, pacemaker spikes will be visible on the EKG strip, but you will note that the pacer spikes are not followed by a QRS complex. Common causes of failure to capture include displacement of lead wire electrodes and battery failure.

Failure of sensing devices in demand pacemakers

Demand pacemakers contain a sensing device. **Sensing** is simply the capability of a pacemaker to recognize inherent electrical activity. If a patient spontaneously develops an adequate heart rate, the demand pacemaker may fail to shut down. If this occurs, the heart's normal heart rate may compete with the rate of the demand pacemaker. In this event, the pacemaker may fire at an inopportune time, such as the vulnerable or relative refractory period during ventricular repolarization, and ventricular fibrillation may ensue. This situation is a dire emergency and must be treated accordingly.

sensing is simply the capability of a pacemaker to recognize inherent electrical conduction system activity

The pacemaker may fail to sense as a result of displacement of the electrode tip, battery failure, lead wire breakage, or significant metabolic variants. Management of a pacemaker that has failed to sense includes correcting the underlying problem.

CLINICAL SIGNIFICANCE OF PACEMAKER RHYTHMS

Under normal circumstances, patients with artificial pacemakers require no unique medical attention. It is critical to note, however, that pacemaker failure produces a life-threatening event in patients whose underlying rhythm is insufficient to maintain cardiac output and adequate systemic perfusion. In these situations, the patient should be immediately transported to a definitive care facility for further intervention.

The vast majority of today's modern artificial pacemakers present no problems. In fact, some of today's pacemakers have dual functions (ICD) in that they not only are capable of pacing the heart, but also recognize certain dysrhythmias and defibrillate, if indicated.

It is also important to note that problems with pacemakers usually occur within the first month after implantation. Occasional problems associated with the implantation procedure may include pneumothorax, induced cardiac dysrhythmias, bleeding, and—very rarely—air embolus.

Whenever you encounter an unconscious patient, you should remember to examine the patient for the presence of a medic alert apparatus, as well as for a small palpable mass underneath the skin in the patient's upper chest or upper abdomen. The presence of either may alert you to the probability of an implanted artificial pacemaker.

Dysrhythmias associated with pacemaker failure are treated the same as dysrhythmias in any other patient. Although patients with pacemakers should be defibrillated like other patients, it is important to note that the defibrillator paddles/pads should not be discharged directly over the battery pack.

CHAPTER 12

 SUMMARY

Artificial pacemakers have the capability to produce an electrical stimulus when the heart's inherent electrical conduction ability is compromised. This is accomplished through the implantation of electrodes within the heart.

These artificial pacemakers are classified as transcutaneous, transvenous, or permanent. Medical science has advanced to the point where problems with pacemakers are rare.

 KEY POINTS TO REMEMBER

1. An artificial pacemaker is an artificial regulator of heart rate.

2. Pacemakers are necessitated when a patient's inherent electrical conduction pathway fails to function sufficiently.

3. Transcutaneous pacing is recommended in the bradycardia algorithm.

4. For the prehospital provider, it is critical to remember that voice contact with medical direction is strongly recommended.

5. Because of various factors, that is, patient movement, the preset heart rate and amperage may need to be adjusted in order to ensure capture.

6. Transvenous pacing is more invasive in nature than TCP.

7. Pacemakers are preset, or programmed, to pace (or deliver electrical impulses) in two modes; fixed rate or demand.

8. Permanent or implanted pacemakers are used with patients who are symptomatic due to bradycardia or complete heart blocks and have not responded to pharmacologic interventions.

9. Remember that properly functioning pacemakers will produce rhythms with pacemaker spikes.

10. It is essential that you recognize that the presence of pacemaker spikes indicates only that the pacemaker is firing and not that mechanical activity is taking place in the myocardium.

11. Common problems associated with pacemakers include battery failure, runaway pacemakers, failure to capture, and failure of sensing devices in demand pacemakers.

 REVIEW QUESTIONS

1. AV sequential pacemakers stimulate only the atria.
   a. False
   b. True

2. _____ is indicated on an EKG strip when there is a P wave or QRS complex following each pacemaker spike.
   a. Sensing
   c. Loss of sensing
   b. Capture
   d. Loss of capture

3. Atrial pacemakers are commonly used today.
   a. True
   b. False

4. The two types of temporary pacemakers include the transvenous pacemaker and the _____ pacemaker.
   a. Ventricular
   c. Transcutaneous
   b. Atrial
   d. Sensing

5. Indications for the use of artificial pacemakers include:
   a. Asymptomatic bradycardia
   b. Symptomatic complete heart block ·
   c. Asymptomatic second-degree heart block
   d. First-degree heart block

6. The EKG wave produced by an artificial pacemaker is referred to as a(n):
   a. Pacemaker spike
   c. Aberration
   b. Ectopic focus
   d. Anomaly

7. The AHA has now recognized the use of transcutaneous pacemaker devices in the bradycardia algorithm.
   a. True
   b. False

8. Ventricular asystole represents an absence of all ventricular electrical activity on an EKG strip.
   a. True
   b. False

9. Symptomatic bradycardia must be confirmed prior to implementing TCP procedures.
   a. True
   b. False

10. Possible problems associated with pacemakers include:
    a. Battery failure
    c. Failure to sense
    b. Failure to capture
    d. All the above

11. Transvenous (through a vein) pacing is another method for delivering electrical impulses to the myocardial tissue.
    a. True
    b. False

12. TCP consists of two large electrode pads, which are most commonly placed in an anterior-posterior or anterior-lateral position on the patient's chest in order to conduct electrical impulses through the skin to the heart.
    a. True
    b. False

13. Under normal circumstances, patients with artificial pacemakers require no unique medical attention.
    a. True
    b. False

14. Dysrhythmias associated with pacemaker failure are treated the same as dysrhythmias in any other patient.
    a. True
    b. False

15. Although patients with pacemakers should be defibrillated like any other patient, it is important to note that the defibrillator paddles/pads should not be discharged directly over the battery pack.
    a. True
    b. False

REVIEW STRIPS

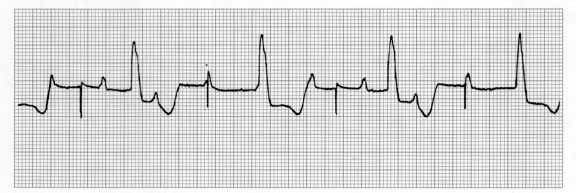

1. Rate _____   Rhythm _____

   P wave _____   PR interval _____

   QRS complex _____   Interpretation _____

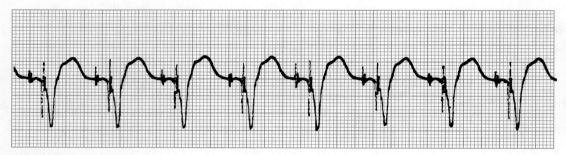

2. Rate _____   Rhythm _____

   P wave _____   PR interval _____

   QRS complex _____   Interpretation _____

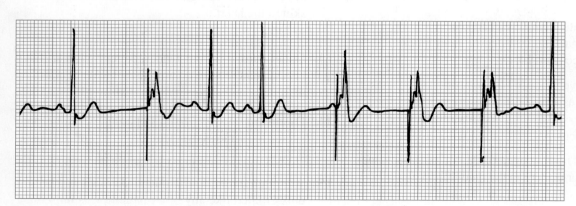

3. Rate _____   Rhythm _____

   P wave _____   PR interval _____

   QRS complex _____   Interpretation _____

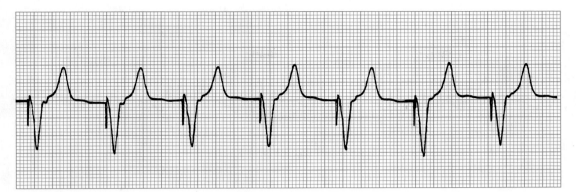

4. Rate _____ Rhythm _____

   P wave _____ PR interval _____

   QRS complex _____ Interpretation _____

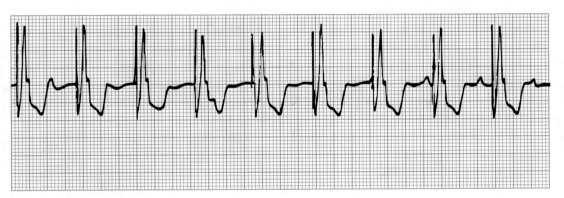

5. Rate _____ Rhythm _____

   P wave _____ PR interval _____

   QRS complex _____ Interpretation _____

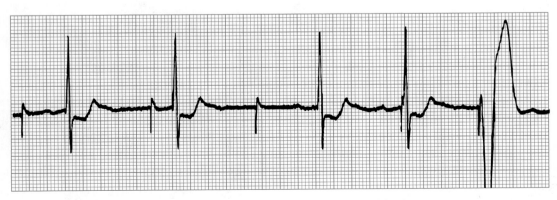

6. Rate _____ Rhythm _____

   P wave _____ PR interval _____

   QRS complex _____ Interpretation _____

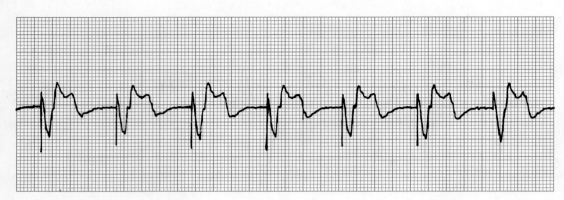

7. Rate _____   Rhythm _____

   P wave _____   PR interval _____

   QRS complex _____   Interpretation _____

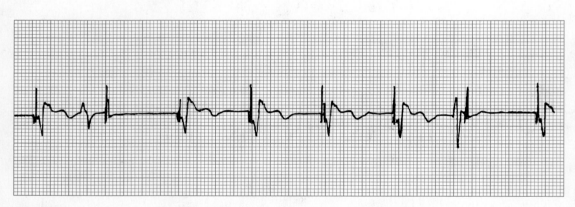

8. Rate _____   Rhythm _____

   P wave _____   PR interval _____

   QRS complex _____   Interpretation _____

Assessment and Treatment of the Patient with Cardiac Emergencies

INTRODUCTION

Cardiac emergencies, including acute myocardial infarction (AMI), continue to be one of the nation's leading causes of death; some of the most recent statistics demonstrate that approximately one in three American adults suffer from one or more types of cardiovascular disease. Heart attacks and other cardiac emergencies affect more than five million individuals each year. More than one million deaths each year are directly attributed to heart disease. Your thorough understanding of the clinical picture of patients who present with cardiac emergencies will enhance your ability to assess and treat these patients in a more time-efficient manner.

CHEST PAIN

Cardiac versus noncardiac

Chest pain of cardiac origin may present in various ways. This type of chest pain may be indicative of serious illness, myocardial ischemia, myocardial injury, or simply stress or exercise-related hypoxia.

Chest pain is the most common presenting symptom of cardiac disease, as well as the most common complaint by patients. Chest pain of cardiac origin is typically described as "crushing" or "squeezing" in nature and is commonly associated with nausea, vomiting, and **diaphoresis** (profuse sweating). The pain is often located substernally and may radiate to the jaw, shoulder, arm, and one or more fingers, most commonly on the left side. (See ■ **Figure 13–1**.)

Chest pain from an acute myocardial infarction may escalate in intensity. Patients may express a feeling of "impending doom" and may exhibit extreme anxiety. A common obstacle to timely intervention by a health care provider dealing with a patient who complains of chest pain is denial. Patients often deny the possibility that they may indeed be experiencing a heart attack, thinking, "It can't happen to me."

It is wise to remember that the patient's description of his discomfort is subjective in nature. Often patients prefer to believe that they are merely experiencing indigestion and that the symptoms will be gone by morning. Unfortunately, it may be the patient rather than the symptoms who is gone by morning. However, with proper public education many lives have been saved that otherwise would have been lost; this is due in large part to the simple fact that many hundreds of laypersons have been certified in the skill of cardiopulmonary resuscitation (CPR).

It should be noted that in special circumstances patients may experience no chest pain at all and may still have sustained a myocardial infarction. This is true primarily in the diabetic patient with advanced **neuropathy** due to destruction of

chest pain is the most common presenting symptom of cardiac disease, as well as the most common complaint by patients

diaphoresis profuse sweating

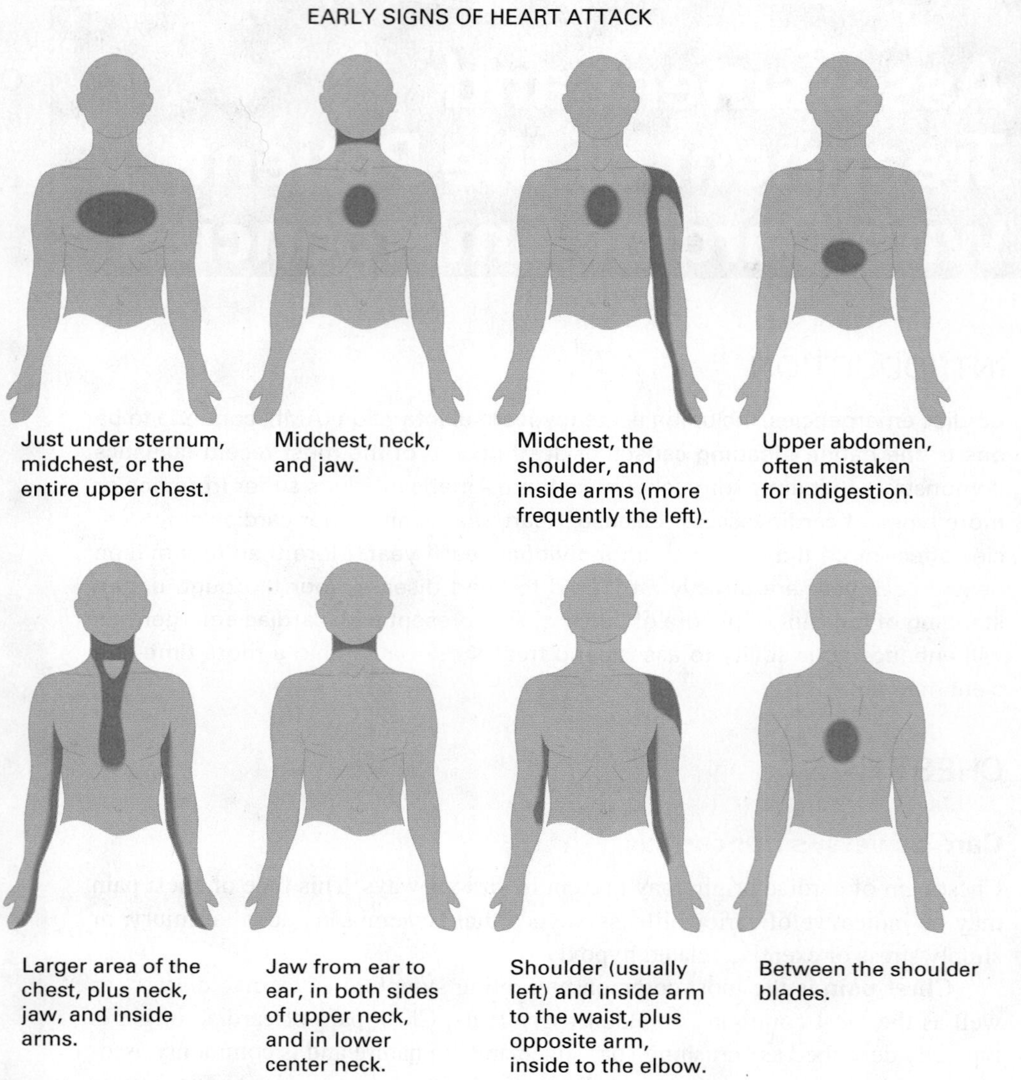

EARLY SIGNS OF HEART ATTACK

Just under sternum, midchest, or the entire upper chest.

Midchest, neck, and jaw.

Midchest, the shoulder, and inside arms (more frequently the left).

Upper abdomen, often mistaken for indigestion.

Larger area of the chest, plus neck, jaw, and inside arms.

Jaw from ear to ear, in both sides of upper neck, and in lower center neck.

Shoulder (usually left) and inside arm to the waist, plus opposite arm, inside to the elbow.

Between the shoulder blades.

FIGURE 13–1. Typical locations and radiation of chest pain associated with cardiac emergencies

nerve endings, causing an inability to perceive pain due to diseases of the nerves. The scenario diabetic patients may present is often congestive heart failure. Females at times will present with atypical signs and symptoms. Some elderly patients may also experience an AMI without chest pain; most commonly their only presenting symptom will be a complaint of profound weakness.

Noncardiac causes of chest pain

of noncardiac chest pain are numerous. However, you should remember that chest
diac in nature until proved otherwise, especially in the prehospital arena.
noncardiac chest pain include (but are not limited to) the following:

ammation of the covering of the lungs (pleura)
—inflammation of the cartilage that connects a rib to the breast bone . . .
wn as the costosternal notch.
es—such as fibromyalgia, rheumatoid arthritis, psoriatic arthritis

Pericarditis—inflammation of the pericardial sac (surrounding the heart)

Myocardial contusion—secondary to chest trauma (high incidence of dysrhythmias)

Sickle cell anemia or infections such as osteomyelitis

Muscle strain—secondary to overstretching of the chest wall muscles

Trauma—secondary to an injury to the chest wall or to organs contained within the chest (or both)

Examples of chest injuries secondary to trauma include the following:

Hemothorax—collection of blood within the pleural cavity

Pneumothorax—the collection of air within the pleural cavity

Hemopneumothorax—collection of blood and air within the pleural cavity

Tension pneumothorax—air trapped in the thoracic cavity without an escape route; pressure builds and affects the lungs, heart, and other vital organs

Chest trauma can produce severe chest pain and may indicate a serious condition that requires immediate intervention. Any patient who exhibits chest pain, regardless of the clinical presentation, should be monitored for possible dysrhythmias. Remember the old adage, *an ounce of prevention . . .* when dealing with chest pain. This adage applies because TIME IS MUSCLE!

ANGINA PECTORIS

Angina pectoris is the most commonly expressed symptom of cardiac chest pain and results from a reduction in blood supply to myocardial tissue. The pain is typically temporary. If blood flow is quickly restored, little or no permanent change or damage may result. Angina is characterized by chest pain or discomfort deep in the sternal area and is often described as heaviness, pressure, "vice-like" tightness, or moderately severe pain. It is quite often mistaken for indigestion. This pain can be referred to the neck, lower jaw, left shoulder, arm, and fingers.

Angina pectoris most often results from narrowed or hardened coronary arterial walls (■ Figure 13–2), commonly caused by **atherosclerosis**. This reduction in blood flow results in a reduced supply of oxygen to cardiac muscle cells.

angina pectoris
pain that results from a reduction in blood supply to myocardial tissue

atherosclerosis
narrowed coronary arterial walls, secondary to fatty deposits

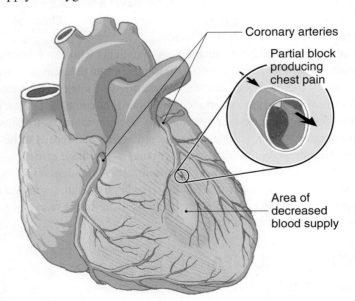

Coronary arteries

Partial block producing chest pain

Area of decreased blood supply

FIGURE 13–2. Partial blockage of a coronary artery deprives an area in the myocardium of oxygen and results in chest pain, or angina pectoris

stable, or predictable angina a particular activity may elicit chest pain

unstable angina pain not elicited by activity that most commonly occurs while the patient is at rest; also referred to as preinfarctional angina

Prinzmetal's angina or vasospastic angina form of angina that can occur when the coronary arteries experience spasms and constrict

The pain is often predictably associated with exercise and is due to the increased pumping activity of the heart, which then requires more oxygen, which the narrowed blood vessels cannot supply. This may be referred to as **stable, or predictable angina**, in that a particular activity may elicit chest pain. The symptoms of stable angina will usually respond well to appropriate treatment, including rest and the administration of oxygen.

Conversely, the pain of **unstable angina** is not elicited by activity and most commonly occurs while the patient is at rest. It is not unusual for these patients to report to you that they were awakened from sleep as a result of significant chest pain. Unstable angina generally indicates a progression of atherosclerotic heart disease and is also referred to as preinfarctional angina.

Yet another form of angina can occur when the coronary arteries experience spasms and constrict, thus significantly decreasing myocardial oxygenation. This type of angina is commonly referred to as **Prinzmetal's angina or vasospastic angina**. It is interesting to note that, in some cases, when a 12-lead EKG is obtained from a patient who is experiencing Prinzmetal's angina, there may be evidence of EKG changes consistent with myocardial injury. However, a 12-lead EKG obtained after nitroglycerin has been administered may illustrate no pattern of injury. In this event, the vasodilation produced by the nitroglycerin alleviated the myocardial ischemia that led to the abnormal EKG. It may be significant to note that although the majority of patients who experience Prinzmetal's angina have underlying atherosclerotic disease, some may have little or none.

Management of the patient who is experiencing angina should center on decreasing the workload of the heart. There are many ways to accomplish this objective, including the following:

- Place the patient at rest in a calm, quiet environment.
- Provide appropriate reassurance to the patient.
- Obtain a 12-lead EKG, if possible.
- Administer oxygen at a high-flow rate in order to increase myocardial oxygenation.
- Establish an intravenous (IV) line to ensure that a lifeline for administration of fluid is available.
- Administer nitroglycerin (per local protocols).

nitroglycerin causes dilation of the blood vessels that consequently reduces the workload of the heart

Nitroglycerin causes dilation of the blood vessels, which consequently reduces the workload of the heart—thus reducing the need for oxygen because the heart has to pump blood against a lesser pressure. The blood tends to remain in the dilated blood vessels, and less blood is returned to the heart for distribution.

An important tool in the diligent management of patients who experience chest pain centers on the necessity of follow-up evaluation. Oftentimes, when the pain goes away, the patient tends to forget that it occurred. Hence, the health care provider must assume the role of patient educator in order to emphasize the importance of further evaluation. Let's face it—if a patient experiences enough pain to cause an ambulance to be summoned or to cause a trip to the emergency department to occur, it stands to reason that this pain needs to be evaluated. We must be diligent and patient, but persistent and persuasive, in these efforts.

A complaint of chest pain should never be minimized. All patients who experience chest pain should be strongly encouraged to be evaluated by a physician. As health care providers we should remember that denial continues to be an obstacle in the care and management of some patients who experience chest pain.

ACUTE MYOCARDIAL INFARCTION

acute myocardial infarction (heart attack) results from a prolonged lack of blood flow to a portion of the myocardial tissue and results in a lack of oxygen

An **acute myocardial infarction (heart attack)** results from a prolonged lack of blood flow to a portion of the myocardial tissue and results in a lack of oxygen. Eventually, myocardial cellular death will follow. Myocardial infarctions vary with the amount of myocardial tissue

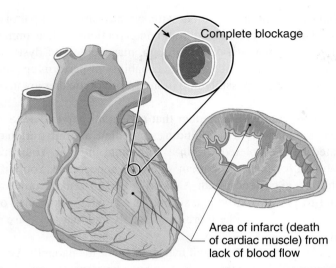

Complete blockage

Area of infarct (death of cardiac muscle) from lack of blood flow

FIGURE 13–3. Complete blockage of a coronary artery will lead to the death of myocardium due to lack of oxygen and to a resulting myocardial infarction

and the portion of the heart affected. If blood supply to cardiac muscle is reestablished within 10 to 20 minutes, there will usually be no permanent injury. If oxygen deprivation lasts longer, cellular death will result. Within 30 to 60 seconds after blockage of a coronary blood vessel, functional changes will become evident. The electrical properties of the cardiac muscle will be altered, and the ability of the cardiac muscle to function properly will be lost.

The most common cause of myocardial infarction is **thrombus formation** that blocks a coronary artery. (See ■ **Figure 13–3**.) Coronary arteries narrowed by atherosclerotic damage are one of the conditions that increase the likelihood of myocardial infarction.

Atherosclerotic lesions partially block blood vessels, resulting in disorderly blood flow, because the surfaces of the lesions are rough. These changes increase the probability of thrombus formation.

thrombus formation the most common cause of myocardial infarction, results in blockage of the coronary artery

Patient assessment and management

In order to assess the patient with chest pain properly, you must be able to recognize the common signs and symptoms. Signs and symptoms of an acute myocardial infarction may be quite similar to those of angina pectoris. Clear differences include the fact that the pain caused by an AMI lasts longer and is usually not relieved by rest. (See ■ **Table 13–1**.)

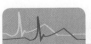 **TABLE 13–1 Differential symptomology: AMI versus angina**

Signs and Symptoms—Angina Pectoris	Signs and Symptoms—Acute Myocardial Infarction
Chest pain: short duration, usually lasts 3–10 min, usually relieved by nitroglycerin	Chest pain: usually lasts more than 2 hrs; not relieved by nitroglycerin
Brought on by stress or exercise and relieved by rest	Usually not precipitated by exercise or stress; not relieved by rest
May be accompanied by dysrhythmias	Usually accompanied by dysrhythmias
Patients usually do not experience nausea, vomiting, or diaphoresis	Patients commonly complain of nausea and vomiting and are often profoundly diaphoretic

The goal of management of the patient with symptomatic chest pain is to interrupt the infarction process. This can be achieved through interventions such as immediate and effective administration of oxygen, alleviation of pain, management of dysrhythmias, efficient and timely transportation to a facility with the capability of performing percutaneous coronary intervention (PCI) and/or possibly initiation of fibrinolytic therapy in order to limit the progression of the infarct.

It is imperative to learn and remember that *time is muscle* and act accordingly. Thus timely assessment and management, including immediate administration of oxygen, must be rapidly initiated and completed within a 10-minute interval. Your initial assessment and evaluation should focus on the patient's general appearance. You will probably note that patients who are experiencing an AMI will tend to remain quiet and still. These patients also tend to prefer a sitting position. The Fowler's or semi-Fowler's position tends to allow the patient to breathe more comfortably and may decrease the workload of the myocardium.

A thorough and timely evaluation and management of the patient's ABCs is imperative. Any problem encountered during this evaluation must be managed quickly and must be followed by a rapid assessment of the vital signs. Because of the wide variations of the presenting vital signs, the clinician should be aware that vital signs are not necessarily reliable in diagnosing an AMI. In spite of this fact, it is important that you monitor and record these signs at frequent intervals.

One of the most important assessment tools that you will use when managing a suspected AMI patient is the cardiac monitor. Dysrhythmias that originate from ischemic and injured myocardial tissues are a common complication of acute myocardial infarctions.

It is critical to understand that in the clinical setting, dysrhythmias may be simply warning signs or may signal severe life-threatening events. In either case, you must not ignore the presence of any abnormal heart rhythm when dealing with a patient who exhibits a "textbook" clinical presentation of an acute myocardial infarction. Although the three-lead (or five-lead) EKG strip will depict the heart rate and rhythm adequately, the 12-lead EKG has the ability to afford a comprehensive picture of the myocardial events occurring during an acute myocardial infarction. For an in-depth discussion relative to 12-lead EKGs, please refer to this book's companion text, *Understanding 12-Lead EKGs: A Practical Approach, 3rd ed.*

Your suspicion of an acute myocardial infarction must be based on the combination of a positive 12-lead EKG and the patient's clinical "picture" (signs and symptoms) in the prehospital arena. Keep in mind that a negative 12-lead EKG does *NOT* rule out the presence of an AMI. Remember also that any patients who complain of chest pain must be thoroughly evaluated, and their management should continue until the possibility of AMI is ruled out by the physician.

oxygen the most important drug that any patient with chest pain can receive

Without a doubt, the most important drug that any patient with chest pain can receive is **oxygen**. Time and again, in this and other textbooks, you will see that statement—simply because it is true and it is critically important to the viability of your patient.

Other considerations regarding treatment include the following:

- Administering oxygen to maintain a saturation of 95 percent or higher.
- Establishing an IV lifeline (according to local protocols)
- Measuring oxygen saturation level (pulse oximetry), if equipment is available
- Continuous cardiac monitoring
- Consider administration of Aspirin (follow local protocols)
- Pain control and management—nitroglycerin, morphine sulfate, and so on (according to local protocols)
- Fibrinolytic therapy and/or Percutaneous Coronary Intervention (PCI)

Remember that the focus of assessment and treatment of the patient who presents with chest pain centers on the immediate oxygenation of hypoxic tissue. Treatment initiatives will vary, depending upon your patient's specific situation; however, you must focus on continual and thorough assessment until such time as the patient is clinically stable.

As mentioned at the beginning of this chapter, cardiac emergencies, including acute myocardial infarction, continue to be one of the nation's leading causes of death. Thus the significance of the patient's condition, as well as the need for early intervention for a patient with suspected AMI, is paramount. An acute myocardial infarction may be a staggering event involving disturbances of the electrical conduction system, as well as mechanical failure secondary to infarcted tissue.

HEART FAILURE

For many years, the term heart failure was considered by many to refer to a singular disease process, most often divided into simply left or right heart failure, but may involve both sides of the heart simultaneously. In more recent years, heart failure, along with all its variations, has been more correctly regarded as a clinical syndrome. **Heart failure** can be simply defined as the inability of the myocardium to pump enough oxygen-rich blood to meet the cardiac output demands of the body. The severity of heart failure depends on how much pumping capacity the heart has lost.

Heart failure may occur from a variety of determinants, including, but not limited to, the following:

heart failure the inability of the myocardium to meet the cardiac output demands of the body

- Coronary disease
- Valvular disease
- Myocardial injury
- Myocarditis

Other clinical symptomologies that may influence heart disease include:

- Dysrhythmias
- Hypertension
- Pulmonary emboli
- Systemic sepsis
- Electrolyte disturbances

Left ventricular failure

When a patient's left ventricle ceases to function in an adequately capacity as to sustain sufficient systemic cardiac output, regardless of the specific cause, this condition is referred to as **left ventricular failure**. In considering the physiology of left heart failure, it is important to recall that blood has been delivered appropriately into the cavity; however, the myocardial musculature of the left ventricle cannot contract sufficiently to empty the blood into the systemic circulation.

left ventricular failure when a patient's left ventricle ceases to function in an adequate capacity to sustain sufficient systemic cardiac output

Common causes of left ventricular failure include, but are not limited to:

Leaking heart valves
Myocardial infarction
Hypertension
Myocarditis
Excessive alcohol intake

As a result of the insufficient emptying of the left ventricle, stroke volume is decreased. When stroke volume is decreased, the body's compensatory mechanisms (increased heart

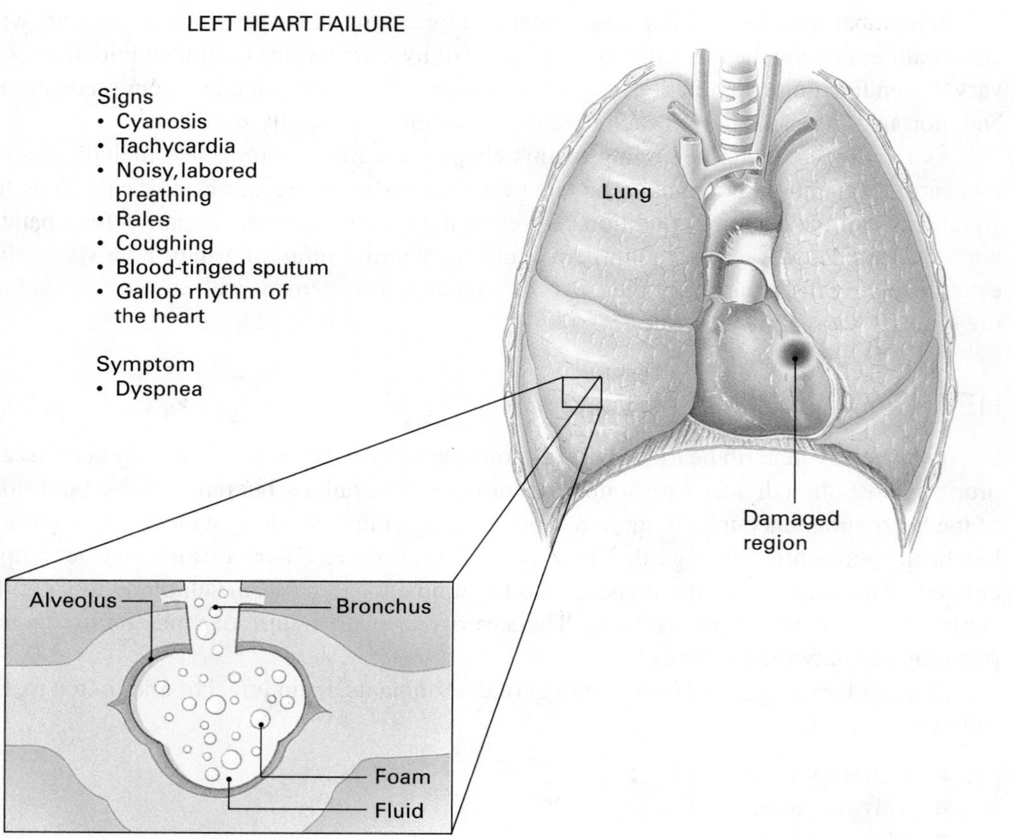

LEFT HEART FAILURE

Signs
- Cyanosis
- Tachycardia
- Noisy, labored breathing
- Rales
- Coughing
- Blood-tinged sputum
- Gallop rhythm of the heart

Symptom
- Dyspnea

FIGURE 13–4. Left heart failure

rate, vasoconstriction, etc.) begin to function at an accelerated rate, in an effort to restore organ perfusion. As a consequence of these mechanisms, pressure in the right as well as the left atrium rises dramatically. It is at this point that the overloaded heart pushes the blood back into the pulmonary system. This backup in the pulmonary system causes plasma to mix with and displace alveolar air, resulting in **pulmonary edema**. This influx of fluid into the alveoli impedes the ability of the alveoli to function properly; thus gas exchange is severely compromised. This compromise, if not corrected promptly, eventually leads to **hypoxia**.

Due to the engorgement of the alveoli, the patient may present with the characteristic symptom of pink, frothy sputum and significant dyspnea. It is important to remember that if left untreated, severe left heart failure can lead to extreme hypoxia and subsequent death.

Emergency management of left heart failure (■ **Figure 13–4**) is aimed at decreasing myocardial oxygen demand, improving myocardial contractility, and improving oxygenation and ventilation. Factors to consider in the treatment and management of left heart failure include these:

■ Allow the patient to assume a position of comfort; if clinically feasible, the patient's legs should be allowed to dangle off the bed or cot.
■ Provide 100 percent high-flow oxygenation via a nonrebreather mask.
■ Utilize pulse oximetry to maintain O_2 saturation of at least 95 percent.
■ Consider the use of CPAP in the presence of pulmonary edema
■ Carefully monitor the patient's LOC for signs of deterioration.
■ Establish an IV line at KVO (keep vein open) rate; carefully restrict intake.

pulmonary edema backup of blood in the pulmonary system that causes plasma to mix with and displace alveolar air

hypoxia low oxygen level

- Establish and maintain EKG monitoring and obtain EKG strip.
- Obtain permission from medical control physician, or follow local protocol for administration of medication (or both).

Medications commonly prescribed to treat the patient experiencing left heart failure include:

- Morphine sulfate
- Furosemide (Lasix)
- Nitroglycerin
- Beta-blockers
- Digitalis

It is imperative to remember that the primary goal of treatment in managing a patient with left heart failure is to ensure adequate oxygenation and to expedite transport to a medical facility.

Right heart failure

When the right ventricle ceases to function properly, this causes an increase in pressure within the right atrium, thus forcing the blood backward into the systemic venous system. It is important to note here that the most common cause of **right heart failure** (■ **Figure 13–5**) is left heart failure. This is because left heart failure produces elevated pressure in the pulmonary vascular system, increasing the workload of the right heart. This backup of pressure

right heart failure when the right ventricle ceases to function properly, causing an increase in pressure within the right atrium, thus forcing the blood backward into the systemic venous system

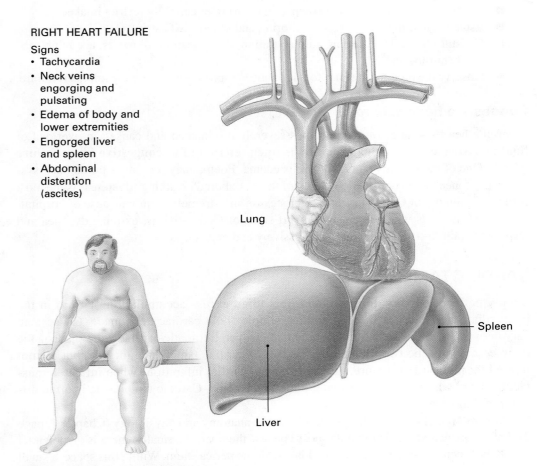

RIGHT HEART FAILURE

Signs
- Tachycardia
- Neck veins engorging and pulsating
- Edema of body and lower extremities
- Engorged liver and spleen
- Abdominal distention (ascites)

Lung

Spleen

Liver

FIGURE 13–5. Right heart failure

forces the plasma into the interstitial tissue, resulting in edema of the lower extremities and sacral area. Subsequently the whole myocardial musculature will weaken, leading to eventual failure of the entire organ.

Often, the terms heart failure and ventricular failure are used interchangeably. Although there are numerous diseases that may precipitate right heart failure, the more common ones include:

- Left heart failure
- Valvular heart disease
- COPD or cor pulmonale
- Pulmonary embolism
- Chronic hypertension

Emergency management of right heart failure is focused primarily on the results of your assessment of the patient. Often patients who are experiencing right heart failure are not considered a medical emergency unless there is associated pulmonary edema or other overt signs of left heart failure. It is important to note that hypotension secondary to right heart failure, which is often seen in right ventricle infarcts, may mimic cardiogenic shock.

Factors to consider in the treatment and management of right heart failure include these:

- Allow the patient to assume a position of comfort; semi-Fowler's is the optimal position.
- Provide oxygenation at the level necessary to maintain saturation of at least 95 percent per pulse oximetry.
- Establish an IV line at KVO (keep vein open) rate; carefully restrict intake.
- Establish and maintain EKG monitoring and obtain EKG strip.
- Consult physician regarding administration of medication (diuretics, ace inhibitors, and beta-blockers).
- Observe the patient carefully for signs and symptoms of developing left heart failure.

Congestive heart failure

When the heart's stroke volume becomes severely diminished and causes an overload of fluid in systemic tissues, this condition is often referred to as **congestive heart failure (CHF)**. One of the primary signs of CHF is edema. Edema may present as pulmonary, systemic, peritoneal, or a combination of any of these. Labored breathing (**dyspnea**) is the most common symptom of CHF. This disease process is an extremely common cause of hospitalization. All patients who present with overt signs of CHF—that is, extreme dyspnea and respiratory failure—must be treated aggressively and expeditiously.

CARDIAC TAMPONADE

Simply defined, **cardiac tamponade** refers to an excess accumulation of fluid in the pericardial sac. However, there is nothing simple about cardiac tamponade. Causes can vary between medical and traumatic events; however, traumatic cardiac tamponade is the more common of the two. Some other causes of cardiac tamponade include, but are not limited to: myocardial rupture, pericarditis, myocardial infarction (when infarcted muscle thins and tears), and blunt force trauma to the chest. Cardiac tamponade is often difficult to diagnose.

You will recall from the discussion of cardiac anatomy and physiology (Chapter 1, page 2) that the **pericardium** is the outermost layer of the heart. Normally, there is a "potential space" between the visceral and parietal layers of the pericardium. Within this space, a small amount of pericardial fluid (approximately 10–20 cc) is present. If, as a result of injury or

congestive heart failure (CHF) when the heart's stroke volume becomes severely diminished and causes an overload of fluid in systemic tissues

dyspnea labored breathing

cardiac tamponade an excess accumulation of fluid in the pericardial sac

pericardium the outermost layer of the heart; potential space between the visceral and parietal layers of the pericardium holds a small amount of pericardial fluid (approximately 10–20 cc)

disease, blood accumulates between the myocardium and pericardium, the ventricles will be compromised. When ventricular filling is impeded, cardiac output falls.

Signs and symptoms of cardiac tamponade include:

- Muffled heart sounds and ST segment changes
- Distention of the jugular vein (JVD)
- Narrowing pulse pressure
- Hypotension (may be extreme)
- Dyspnea
- Weak, rapid pulse

Sometimes referred to as **Beck's triad**, muffled heart sounds, JVD, and narrowing pulse pressure are commonly called the "classic" indicators of cardiac tamponade. A **pulsus paradoxus**, as evidenced by a systolic blood pressure that drops more than 10 to 15 mmHg during inspiration, may also occur with cardiac tamponade.

Emergency management of cardiac tamponade includes the following:

- Prompt recognition
- Ensure and maintain a patent airway.
- Administer 100 percent high-flow oxygen.
- Monitor pulse oximetry—maintain O_2 saturation of 95 percent.
- Establish and maintain IV support.
- Administer pharmacological agents as indicated.
- Transport expeditiously.

The therapy of choice involves intervention by the physician, in most instances. Called a pericardiocentesis, this invasive procedure consists of aspiration of fluid from the pericardium with a needle. Remember, cardiac tamponade is a true medical emergency. If the patient is to survive this dire condition, the pericardial blood must be removed and the source of bleeding stopped.

CARDIOGENIC SHOCK

When left ventricular function is so severely compromised that the heart can no longer meet the metabolic requirements of the body, **cardiogenic shock** may occur. This condition is often a result of extensive myocardial infarction and is said to be the most critical form of heart failure. Ineffective myocardial contractions result in a marked decrease in stroke volume, as well as significantly decreased cardiac output, ultimately leading to inadequate tissue perfusion.

The onset of cardiogenic shock may be abrupt or gradual; however, many and varied causes have been identified. These causes can relate to interference with myocardial contractility, preload, or afterload. Causes may also be related to **hypovolemia** or various pathophysiological disorders, dysrhythmias, and cardiomyopathy.

Trauma-related injuries that result in cardiac tamponade, tension pneumothorax, or both can compress the myocardium and produce severe compromise in ventricular filling. Severe pulmonary embolism may contribute to poor ventricular emptying.

Cardiogenic shock is most often associated with large anterior infarctions, as well as those that involve loss of more than 40 percent of the left ventricle. The mortality rate following episodes of cardiogenic shock is high, especially when dealing with geriatric patients.

Assessment of the patient in cardiogenic shock will focus on identifying the cause. Signs and symptoms will vary widely and will be based on the specific causative factor. As with all patients, it is imperative that you recognize and treat any life-threatening problems. You should also closely monitor the patient's level of consciousness, being especially

Beck's triad muffled heart sounds, JVD, and narrowing pulse pressure

pulsus paradoxus evidenced by a systolic blood pressure that drops more than 10 to 15 mmHg during inspiration

cardiogenic shock when left ventricular function is so severely compromised that the heart can no longer meet the metabolic requirements of the body

hypovolemia decreased blood volume

attentive to alterations in mental status. In addition, an adequate patient history, if obtainable, may prove to be helpful to the patient's attending physician.

Patients in cardiogenic shock will often present with signs and symptoms of myocardial infarction. These symptoms may quickly deteriorate to manifestation of clinical evidence of severe systemic hypoperfusion. The manifestations may include:

- Profound hypotension (systolic BP usually less than 80 mmHg)
- Compensatory tachycardia
- Tachypnea, often resulting from associated pulmonary edema
- Cool, clammy skin caused by massive vasoconstriction
- Major dysrhythmias
- Respiratory difficulty
- Peripheral edema
- Pulmonary edema

Management of cardiogenic shock must be aggressive. Patients who are in cardiogenic shock should be considered seriously ill. If the patient presents in the prehospital arena, rapid transport should be quickly facilitated.

Immediate management of the patient in cardiogenic shock should be based upon the patient's clinical presentation. You should be attentive to identifying and treating the underlying cause or causes of the patient's signs and symptoms. If the patient is conscious, take care to maintain a calm demeanor and reassure the patient and his or her family.

Aggressive treatment measures may include:

- Airway management and ventilatory support, including administration of high-flow oxygen
- Consider the use of CPAP in the presence of pulmonary edema
- Circulatory support, including IV therapy
- Allowing the patient to assume a position of comfort, if clinically feasible
- EKG monitoring and treatment of presenting dysrhythmias
- Frequent evaluation of vital signs
- Pulse oximetry, to maintain O_2 saturation at 95 percent or better
- Medication therapy, including various vasopressors, such as dopamine, dobutamine, and Levophed, as well as morphine sulfate, nitroglycerin, Lasix, and/or digitalis

Remember that cardiogenic shock has a relatively high mortality rate; thus the patient must be treated aggressively and immediately. You should identify and treat the underlying cause of the patient's problem and transport the patient expeditiously.

CHAPTER 13

 SUMMARY

Patients who experience chest pain account for the majority of all EMS calls in this country. Thousands of Americans die each year from cardiovascular emergencies, and many of these deaths occur in the prehospital arena. Cardiovascular emergencies are primarily related to obstruction of the coronary arteries due to spasm or thrombus. As health care providers, we must be able to recognize the warning signs of various cardiovascular emergencies. In addition, we must be able to intervene with appropriate and timely management.

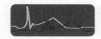

KEY POINTS TO REMEMBER

1. The most common presenting symptom of cardiac disease is chest pain; however, you must remember that chest pain is cardiac in nature until proven otherwise!

2. Chest pain is typically described as crushing or squeezing and is associated with other symptoms, such as nausea, vomiting, and diaphoresis.

3. Some patients (particularly the elderly, females, and diabetic) will have an atypical presentation due to neuropathy and will not present with chest pain as their main symptom or complaint.

4. Pain that results from ischemia due to a reduction of blood supply to myocardial tissue is termed angina pectoris.

5. Angina is typically temporary and stops when O_2 demand decreases.

6. The narrowing and hardening of the coronary arteries most often caused by fatty deposits and reduces blood supply is called atherosclerosis.

7. The main pharmacologic intervention in angina is the drug nitroglycerin.

8. Nitroglycerin dilates the coronary arteries and reduces workload of the heart.

9. Lack of oxygen to the myocardial tissue may result in a myocardial infarction.

10. The most common cause of myocardial infarction is thrombus formation either at the site of narrowing in a coronary artery or a thrombus forming somewhere else and traveling into the narrowed artery.

11. The term *time is muscle* is imperative for the practitioner to understand in that the more time it takes to correct the blockage, the more muscle that is damaged.

12. In the treatment modalities of myocardial infarction, OXYGEN is the most important drug that must be given to the patient.

13. Oxygen is then followed by nitroglycerin, morphine, and the consideration of fibrinolytic therapy; however, PCI preferred.

14. The inability of the myocardium to meet cardiac output demands to the body is termed heart failure and can be subdivided into left heart failure (LHF) and right heart failure (RHF), depending on the symptoms elicited.

15. LHF develops when a patient's left ventricle ceases to function in an adequate capacity as to sustain sufficient systemic cardiac output.

16. RHF may occur when the right ventricle ceases to function properly, causing an increase in pressure within the right atrium, thus forcing the blood backward into the systemic venous system.

17. When there is fluid buildup in the pericardial sac, this is termed cardiac tamponade and is potentially deadly unless reversed.

18. When systolic blood pressure drops more than 10 to 15 mmHg during inspiration, this condition is termed pulsus paradoxus and is an indicator of cardiac tamponade.

19. Cardiogenic shock develops when the capability of the ventricular myocardial musculature is so severely compromised that the heart no longer meets the metabolic demands of the body.

20. Cardiogenic shock has a relatively high mortality rate and must be treated aggressively and immediately.

REVIEW QUESTIONS

1. A common obstacle to the timely intervention by a health care provider when a patient complains of chest pain is:
   a. Mistrust
   b. Timidity
   c. Anxiety
   d. Denial

2. Collateral circulation allows for:
   a. Alternative path of blood flow in the event of occlusion
   b. Circulation continuum during diastole
   c. Maintaining artery patency during spasms
   d. Blood flow continuum during systole

3. The pain of angina pectoris:
   a. Is always constant
   b. Is typically temporary
   c. Occurs only during rest
   d. Is never mistaken for indigestion

4. Myocardial infarction is:
   a. Always temporary
   b. Usually diagnosed within 24 hours
   c. Age-limited in most patients
   d. Due to myocardial cell death

5. The most common cause of AMIs is:
   a. Coronary vasospasms
   b. Atherosclerotic lesions
   c. Thrombus formation
   d. Arteriosclerotic blebs

6. In acute myocardial infarctions, chest pain is:
   a. Short in duration and relieved by nitroglycerin
   b. Short in duration but not relieved by nitroglycerin
   c. Long in duration and relieved by nitroglycerin
   d. Long in duration and not relieved by nitroglycerin

7. Patients experiencing an acute myocardial infarction will always complain of chest pain.
   a. True
   b. False

8. Some elderly patients may experience an AMI without chest pain; most commonly their only presenting symptom will be a complaint of profound:
   a. Depression
   b. Weakness
   c. Nausea
   d. Dizziness

9. Unstable angina generally indicates progression of atherosclerotic heart disease and is also referred to as:
   a. PND
   b. Cor pulmonale
   c. Infarctional angina
   d. Preinfarctional angina

10. When interpreting dysrhythmias, you should remember that the most important key is the:
    a. PR interval
    b. Rate and rhythm
    c. Presence of dysrhythmias
    d. Patient's clinical appearance

11. The primary goal of management of the patient with symptomatic chest pain is to:
    a. Interrupt the infarction process
    b. Augment the infarction process
    c. Institute fibrinolytic therapy
    d. Increase myocardial oxygen consumption

12. Management of a patient who is suspected of having sustained a myocardial contusion should:
    a. Focus primarily on the associated and isolated chest injury
    b. Be similar to the treatment administered to a suspected MI patient
    c. Be initiated only at the definitive care facility following transport
    d. Be completed in the prehospital arena, before transport to the hospital

13. Emergency management of left heart failure is aimed at:
    a. Decreasing myocardial oxygen demand
    b. Improving myocardial contractility
    c. Improving oxygenation and ventilation
    d. All the above

14. Medications commonly prescribed to treat the patient experiencing left heart failure include:
    a. Adenosine
    b. Prednisone
    c. Heparin
    d. Furosemide

15. It is important to note that hypotension secondary to right heart failure, which is often seen in right ventricle infarcts, may mimic:
    a. Angina pectoris
    b. Pneumothorax
    c. Cardiogenic shock
    d. Neurogenic shock

16. Signs and symptoms of cardiac tamponade include all the following except:
    a. Muffled heart sounds
    b. Jugular vein distention
    c. Widening pulse pressure
    d. Hypotension

17. A pulsus paradoxus, as evidenced by a systolic blood pressure that drops more than _____ mmHg during inspiration, may occur in cardiac tamponade.
    a. 20–25   c. 25–30
    b. 10–15   d. 35–40

18. When ineffective myocardial contractions result in a marked decrease in stroke volume, as well as significantly decreased cardiac output, ultimately leading to inadequate tissue perfusion, this condition is known as _____ shock.
    a. Cardiogenic
    b. Neurogenic
    c. Psychogenic
    d. Hypovolemic

19. Cardiogenic shock is most often associated with large infarctions, as well as those that involve loss of more than 40 percent of the left _____ ventricle.
    a. Inferior   c. Anterior
    b. Posterior   d. Lateral

20. Patients in cardiogenic shock will often present with signs and symptoms of myocardial infarction.
    a. True   b. False

14

More Review Questions

1. The majority of all cardiac dysrhythmias are caused by ischemia secondary to hypoxia; therefore, the most appropriate drug to give a patient with any dysrhythmia is:
   - **a.** Oxygen
   - **b.** D5W
   - **c.** Lidocaine
   - **d.** Morphine

2. The fibrous sac, covering the outer layer of the heart, which is in contact with the pleura, is the:
   - **a.** Epicardium
   - **b.** Myocardium
   - **c.** Pericardium
   - **d.** Endocardium

3. The lower chamber of the heart, that is, the ventricle with the thicker myocardium is the:
   - **a.** Right
   - **b.** Left

4. The pulmonic and aortic valves, which allow blood flow to the pulmonary and systemic circulation, are open during:
   - **a.** Systole
   - **b.** Diastole

5. The large blood vessel that returns unoxygenated blood from the head and neck to the right atrium is called the:
   - **a.** Jugular vein
   - **b.** Carotid artery
   - **c.** Superior vena cava
   - **d.** Inferior vena cava

6. The coronary sinus, also referred to as the Great Cardiac vein, which opens into the right atrium, allows venous return from the:
   - **a.** Azygos
   - **b.** Pleura
   - **c.** Myocardium
   - **d.** Endocardium

7. The sawtooth pattern is indicative of which rhythm?
   - **a.** Atrial fibrillation
   - **b.** Atrial asystole
   - **c.** Ventricular flutter
   - **d.** Atrial flutter

8. The mitral valve, sometimes referred to as the bicuspid, is located between the:
   - **a.** Right and left atrium
   - **b.** Right and left ventricle
   - **c.** Left atrium and left ventricle
   - **d.** Right atrium and right ventricle

9. The QRS waves of all premature complexes are usually 0.10 seconds or less.
   - **a.** False
   - **b.** True

10. The most appropriate initial w/s for defibrillating ventricular fibrillation with a monophasic defibrillator in an adult is:
    - **a.** 400 Joules
    - **b.** 360 Joules
    - **c.** 1 Joule per kilogram
    - **d.** 20–25 Joules per kilogram

11. When preparing to defibrillate a patient who presents with ventricular fibrillation, the health care provider should do all the following except:
    a. Check pulses and lead wires
    b. Order all personnel to stand clear
    c. Perform cardiopulmonary resuscitation
    d. Ensure that the synchronization button is on

12. The most appropriate treatment of uncomplicated acute myocardial infarction is:
    a. IV D5W, Nitroglycerine
    b. Oxygen by mask, IV LR
    c. IV NS, monitor, O_2
    d. IV D5W, monitor O_2

13. The coronary arteries arise from the trunk of the _____ and function to carry oxygenated blood throughout the myocardium:
    a. Aorta
    b. Coronary sinus
    c. Pulmonary veins
    d. Pulmonary arteries

14. In the prehospital field, we administer IV fluid to a cardiac patient in order to:
    a. Provide a lifeline
    b. Allow oxygen to reach the brain
    c. Keep the patient well hydrated
    d. Prevent incipient pump failure

15. The heart contains four chambers; the chambers that are thin walled and pump against low pressure are the:
    a. Apex
    b. Aorta
    c. Atria
    d. Ventricles

16. Blood pressure (BP) is one of the primary vital signs that is assessed in every patient encounter and is maintained by cardiac output and:
    a. Alveoli perfusion
    b. Stroke volume
    c. Coronary arteries
    d. Peripheral resistance

17. One component of the electrical conduction system, the sinoatrial (SA) node, is located in the:
    a. Right atrium
    b. Right ventricle
    c. Purkinje fiber tract
    d. Atrioventricular septum

18. The atrioventricular (AV) node is located in the:
    a. Right ventricle
    b. Left ventricle
    c. Purkinje fiber tract
    d. Floor of the right atrium

19. The intrinsic firing rate of the AV node is _____ beats per minute (BPM).
    a. 60–100
    b. 25–35
    c. 35–45
    d. 40–60

20. The intrinsic firing rate of the SA node in the adult is _____ BPM.
    a. 20–60
    b. 40–80
    c. 60–100
    d. 80–100

21. The electrocardiogram is a diagnostic tool that is utilized to:
    a. Determine pulse rate
    b. Detect valvular dysfunction
    c. Evaluate electrical activity in the heart
    d. Determine whether the heart muscle is contracting

22. The PR interval represents the time interval necessary for the impulse to travel from the SA node to the AV node and should normally be _____ seconds.
    a. 0.01–0.10
    b. 0.02–0.12
    c. 0.08–0.12
    d. 0.12–0.20

23. The QRS interval represents the conduction of the electrical impulse from the Bundle of His throughout the ventricular muscle and should normally be _____ seconds or smaller.
    a. 0.20
    b. 0.12
    c. 0.18
    d. 0.36

24. The heart has four chambers, two upper chambers and two lower chambers; the upper chambers are called:
    a. Atria
    b. Ventricles
    c. Septa
    d. Branches

25. A sinus rhythm with cyclic variation caused by alterations in the respiratory pattern is:
    a. Sinus arrest
    b. Sinus tachycardia
    c. Sinus dysrhythmia
    d. Supraventricular dysrhythmia

26. A sudden (paroxysmal) onset of tachycardia with a stimulus that arises above the AV node refers to a:
    a. Sinus arrest
    b. Sinus tachycardia
    c. Sinus dysrhythmia
    d. Supraventricular dysrhythmia

27. Oscilloscopic evidence of ventricular fibrillation can be mimicked by artifact.
    a. True
    b. False

28. In the presence of the lethal cardiac dysrhythmia ventricular fibrillation, attempts at countershock might be ineffective because of:
    a. Metabolic acidosis
    b. Ventricular irritability
    c. Inadequate oxygenation
    d. All the above

29. In the presence of a supraventricular tachycardiac (SVT) rhythm, before performing carotid sinus massage, you should do all the following except:
    a. Monitor the EKG
    b. Ensure that the carotid pulses are present
    c. Have the patient perform Valsalva's maneuver
    d. Establish a secure airway by intubating the trachea

30. As a component of the electrical conduction system, the QRS complex is produced when the:
    a. Ventricles repolarize
    b. Ventricles depolarize
    c. Ventricles contract
    d. Both b and c

31. Most atrial fibrillation waveforms are not followed by a QRS complex because the:
    a. Impulses are initiated in the left ventricle
    b. Stimuli are not strong enough to be conducted
    c. Ventricle can receive only 120 stimuli in 1 minute
    d. AV junction is unable to conduct all the excitation impulses

32. Identify the normal impulse flow of the heart's electrical conduction system:
    1. SA node
    2. Purkinje fibers
    3. Bundle of His
    4. AV node

5. Bundle branches
6. Internodal pathways
    a. 1, 5, 2, 4, 6, 3
    b. 1, 6, 4, 3, 5, 2
    c. 1, 4, 3, 6, 5, 2
    d. 1, 2, 3, 4, 5, 6

33. When the cardiac rhythm displayed on the EKG strip shows no relationship between the P wave and the QRS complex, you should suspect:
    a. First-degree block
    b. Second-degree block
    c. Third-degree block
    d. Electromechanical dissociation

34. In the presence of stable angina pectoris, which is often associated with exercise and due to increased oxygen requirements, the pain is most often:
    a. Predictable
    b. Not predictable
    c. Never very severe
    d. Usually undetectable

35. Signs and symptoms that may be observed in a patient with necrotic heart tissue could include all of the following except:
    a. Dysrhythmias
    b. Congestive heart failure
    c. Cardiogenic shock (severe)
    d. Dysphasia

36. The term supraventricular indicates a stimulus arising above the ventricles.
    a. True
    b. False

37. Second-degree heart block, Mobitz type I (or Wenckebach) differs from complete heart block in that CHB has a:
    a. Faster rate
    b. Normal QRS
    c. Constant PR interval
    d. Regular R-R interval

38. Paroxysmal Atrial Tachycardia is a sudden onset of atrial tachycardia.
    a. True
    b. False

39. The T wave represented on an EKG rhythm strip represents:
    a. Rest period
    b. Bundle of His
    c. Atrial contraction
    d. Ventricular contraction

40. Oxygenated blood is distributed throughout the heart muscle through the process known as coronary circulation. The coronary circulation has how many main arteries?
    a. Two
    b. Six
    c. Four
    d. Eight

41. Starling's law may be expressed as follows:
    a. An increase in systolic filling does not alter cardiac output.
    b. A decrease in systolic filling will decrease the force of contraction.
    c. An increase in diastolic filling will increase the force of contraction.
    d. An increase in filling time yields greater cardiac output regardless of peripheral resistance.

42. PEA, or pulseless electrical activity, may be manifested by a(n):
    a. Normal EKG, normal pulse
    b. Normal EKG, absent pulse
    c. Abnormal EKG, normal pulse
    d. Abnormal EKG, absent pulse

43. The function of the chordae tendineae and papillary muscles is to:
    a. Prevent backflow of blood into the ventricles
    b. Protect the coronary orifices when the aortic valve opens
    c. Prevent backflow of blood into the atrium
    d. Facilitate backflow of blood from the aorta

44. A 50-year-old man is complaining of chest pain that began while he was clearing underbrush on a vacant lot. He describes the pain as a "heavy pressure" that has lasted 5 to 10 minutes. Vital signs are: BP = 140/95, pulse = 82, respirations = 16. He has no previous cardiac history. EKG shows Normal Sinus Rhythm. The chest pain is most likely due to:

    a. Dysrhythmias   **c.** Coronary insufficiency

    b. Pulmonary embolus   **d.** Congestive heart failure

45. In the electrocardiograph, Lead II is most commonly used in the prehospital arena because it:

    a. Is easier to apply   **c.** Illustrates good P waves

    b. Shows good T waves   **d.** Is faster to apply

46. Cardiac cells have four primary cell characteristics. One of these properties is the ability of certain cardiac cells to initiate excitation impulses spontaneously and is called:

    a. Automaticity   **c.** Conductivity

    b. Contractility   **d.** Excitability

47. The keys to interpretation of Second-degree heart block, Mobitz type II, are the presence of constant PR intervals and the fact that there are more P waves present than QRS complexes.

    a. True   **b.** False

48. The absence of electrical impulses results in the recording of a flat line on an EKG strip. This rhythm is known as asystole.

    a. False   **b.** True

49. Your patient is a driver who was in a head-on automobile collision. Upon arrival at the patient's side, you immediately notice that the steering wheel is bent and that the patient has multiple contusions on the chest area. You realize you are probably dealing with:

    a. Angina pectoris   **c.** Myocardial trauma

    b. A drunk patient   **d.** Hypertensive crisis

50. A man complains of substernal chest pain radiating to his left arm and jaw. He reports that he has vomited once and continues to feel nauseated. He is sitting upright, appears to be short of breath, and is sweating profusely. Your patient's symptoms most probably are related to:

    a. Pacemaker failure   **c.** Hypertensive crisis

    b. Pulmonary edema   **d.** Acute myocardial infarction

51. If a known coronary bypass patient experiences a cardiac arrest, the health care provider should:

    a. Not perform CPR because of the risk of further injury

    b. Deliver lighter compressions because of the risk of further injury

    c. Provide CPR in the same manner as for any other patient in arrest

    d. Provide CPR unless fracture of the sternum or ribs becomes apparent

52. The expected rate of a junctional escape rhythm is _____ BPM.

    a. 20–40   **c.** 40–60

    b. 60–100   **d.** 60–80

53. When interpreting dysrhythmias, you must always remember that the most important key is the:
- **a.** PR interval
- **b.** Rate and rhythm
- **c.** Presence of dysrhythmias
- **d.** Patient's clinical appearance

54. In order to obtain a Lead II EKG strip, you could, dependent on manufacturer of the monitor, apply any of the following number of leads to the patient's chest except.
- **a.** Three
- **b.** Four
- **c.** Five
- **d.** Six

55. When considering cardiac anatomy, you should realize that the uppermost portion of the heart is known as the:
- **a.** Apex
- **b.** Base
- **c.** Atria
- **d.** Aorta

56. The most common causes of poor electrocardiogram tracings are:
- **a.** Patient movement
- **b.** Loose leads/electrodes
- **c.** Both a and b
- **d.** None of the above

57. "A graphic record of the electrical activity of the heart" describes a(n):
- **a.** Echocardiogram
- **b.** Electrocardiogram
- **c.** Encephalogram
- **d.** Radiogram

58. Premature ventricular contractions (PVCs) with different morphologies are called multifocal PVCs. The primary treatment for multifocal PVCs is:
- **a.** Defibrillation
- **b.** Cardioversion
- **c.** Oxygen administration
- **d.** Lidocaine drip

59. In order to calculate heart rate accurately by the R-to-R interval method, the patient must have a regular rhythm.
- **a.** True
- **b.** False

60. Second-degree heart block, Mobitz Type I, may be transient and self-correcting.
- **a.** True
- **b.** False

61. Cardiovascular disease remains the number one cause of death in the United States.
- **a.** False
- **b.** True

62. Prompt, definitive intervention has proved effective in preventing many deaths from cardiovascular disease.
- **a.** True
- **b.** False

63. The innermost lining of the heart is contiguous with the visceral pericardium and is called the:
- **a.** Endocardium
- **b.** Pericardium
- **c.** Myocardium
- **d.** Epicardium

64. When discussing the anatomy of the heart, you should understand that the right and left atria are separated anatomically by the:
- **a.** Interatrial septum
- **b.** Bundle of Kent
- **c.** Interventricular septum
- **d.** Endocardial mass

65. When considering cardiac anatomy, you recognize that the right atrium receives blood from the myocardium via the:
- **a.** Left marginal branch
- **b.** Inferior vena cava
- **c.** Great cardiac vein
- **d.** Internal carotid artery

66. Two examples of atrioventricular valves are:
    1. Pulmonic valve
    2. Tricuspid valve
    3. Papillary valve
    4. Bicuspid valve
       a. 1 and 2
       b. 2 and 4
       c. 1 and 3
       d. 3 and 4

67. When considering blood return from the systemic and pulmonary circulations, recall that deoxygenated blood enters the heart through the:
    1. Coronary sinus
    2. Pulmonary vein
    3. Superior vena cava
    4. Inferior vena cava
       a. 1, 2, and 3
       b. 2, 3, and 4
       c. 2 and 3 only
       d. 1, 3, and 4

68. In EKG strips representing dysrhythmias originating in the AV junction, the P wave, if present, will be inverted or absent.
    a. True   b. False

69. The amount of blood ejected by the heart in one complete cardiac contraction is known as:
    a. Preload   c. Cardiac cycle
    b. Afterload   d. Stroke volume

70. The pressure in the ventricle at the end of diastole is referred to as:
    a. Preload   c. Cardiac output
    b. Afterload   d. Autonomic

71. The parasympathetic nervous system is mediated by the tenth cranial nerve, which runs from the brain stem to the rectum. This nerve is called the:
    a. Optic   c. Plexus
    b. Vagus   d. Ganglia

72. The neurotransmitter for the parasympathetic nervous system is acetylcholine. Release of acetylcholine:
    1. Slows the heart rate
    2. Increases the heart rate
    3. Slows atrioventricular conduction
    4. Increases atrioventricular conduction
       a. 1 and 3
       b. 2 and 3
       c. 3 and 4
       d. 1 and 4

73. Hyperkalemia refers to an increased level of potassium in the blood and can result in decreased automaticity and conduction.
    a. True   b. False

74. Cardiac function, both electrical and mechanical, is strongly influenced by electrolyte imbalance.
    a. True　　　　　　　　　　　　　b. False

75. An EKG strip illustrates a regular rhythm, a heart rate of 70 BPM, and QRS complexes that are within normal limits. P waves are variable in configuration across the strip. This rhythm is identified as a:
    a. Wandering atrial pacemaker
    b. First-degree heart block
    c. Third-degree heart block
    d. Second-degree heart block, Mobitz I

76. Evidence of ventricular irritability, such as the occurrence of PVCs, in the presence of myocardial infarction is:
    a. A precursor to respiratory involvement
    b. Very dangerous and should be treated
    c. To be expected and not a cause for alarm
    d. Highly unlikely if oxygen is administered

77. Prolonged episodes of SVT may increase myocardial oxygen demand and may thus increase the need for supplemental oxygen therapy.
    a. True　　　　　　　　　　　　　b. False

78. While observing a patient's cardiac monitor, you notice a progressing PR interval until such time that a QRS is dropped. This is considered to be:
    a. Third-degree block
    b. Atrial fibrillation
    c. Second-degree AV block, Mobitz type I
    d. Second-degree AV block, Mobitz type II

79. Artifact can mimic certain lethal dysrhythmias and is defined as EKG waveforms produced from sources outside the heart.
    a. True　　　　　　　　　　　　　b. False

80. Parasympathetic stimulation controls cardiac action by reducing the heart rate, the speed of impulse through the AV node, and the force of atrial contraction. This response is known as the:
    a. Nodal response　　　　　　　c. Neurotransmitter
    b. SA node　　　　　　　　　　　d. Vagal response

81. A cardiac abnormality in the electrical conduction through the ventricles may be identified on the EKG tracing by a(n):
    a. Distorted, varying P wave pattern
    b. Prolonged PR interval
    c. Wide and bizarre QRS complex
    d. Elevated S-T segment

82. All the following statements regarding premature ventricular complexes (PVCs) are true except:
    a. Occasional PVCs may occur in persons without heart disease
    b. Bursts of two or more PVCs in a row may progress rapidly to ventricular tachycardia
    c. A PVC that falls on or near a T wave may cause ventricular fibrillation
    d. Frequent PVCs in a patient without heart disease require no treatment

83. Amiodarone/Lidocaine should be considered for suppressing premature ventricular contractions (PVCs) in acute myocardial infarction in which situation?
    a. When the PVCs are more frequent than six per minute or are multifocal
    b. In the event of second- or third-degree heart block
    c. In the presence of acute onset sinus bradycardia
    d. With a patient who is known to be allergic to local anesthetics

84. The term for the condition in which there are regular ventricular complexes on the EKG monitor but no palpable pulse is:
    a. Pacemaker rhythm
    b. Vagal response
    c. Mechanical CPR
    d. Pulseless electrical activity

85. The pause following an ectopic beat where the SA node is unaffected and the cadence of the heart is uninterrupted is called:
    a. Asynchronous
    b. Noncompensatory
    c. Interpolated
    d. Compensatory

86. The faster discharging rate of the AV junction in an accelerated junctional rhythm may be due to:
    a. Increased automaticity of the AV junction
    b. Blockage of the parasympathetic nervous system response
    c. Increased excitation of the internodal pathways
    d. Increased excitation of the sinoatrial node

87. Paroxysmal junctional tachycardia is often more appropriately called paroxysmal supraventricular tachycardia, since it may be difficult to distinguish this rhythm from paroxysmal atrial tachycardia due to the rapid rate.
    a. True
    b. False

88. Vagal maneuvers such as carotid sinus massage are commonly used to treat symptomatic:
    a. Ventricular tachycardia
    b. Paroxysmal junctional tachycardia
    c. Paroxysmal supraventricular tachycardia
    d. Only b and c

89. All the following are true of third-degree atrioventricular block except:
    a. The atria and the ventricles pace the heart independent of each other
    b. Both the atrial and the ventricular rates are usually regular
    c. There is no relationship between the P waves and the R waves
    d. Although the atria and ventricles are disassociated, their rates are generally the same

90. Defibrillation is the process of passing an electrical current through a fibrillating heart to depolarize the cells and is the treatment of choice for:
    1. Asystole
    2. Pulseless ventricular tachycardia
    3. Ventricular fibrillation
    4. Idioventricular rhythms
        a. 1, 2, and 3
        b. 2 and 3
        c. 1, 3, and 4
        d. 3 and 4

91. A ventricular escape beat or ventricular escape rhythm results when:
  1. The vagus nerve is hyperstimulated
  2. Impulses from higher pacemakers fail to reach the ventricles
  3. A ventricular excitation impulse escapes from the AV junction
  4. The rate of discharge of higher pacemakers becomes less than that of the ventricles
    a. 1 and 3
    b. 2 and 4
    c. 1, 2, and 3
    d. 2, 3, and 4

92. Since unifocal PVCs imply uniform irritability of the entire myocardium, they are generally considered more life-threatening than multifocal PVCs.
    a. True   **b.** False

93. A 69-year-old man is complaining of mild chest pain, and he states that the pain is "traveling down my left arm." Physical exam reveals no other significant findings. Vital signs are: BP = 160/88, pulse = 94 and irregular, respirations = 24. The cardiac monitor reveals a normal sinus rhythm with five unifocal PVCs per minute. The most appropriate prehospital treatment is:
    a. Monitor patient only—no treatment necessary
    b. Oxygen at 4 L per nasal cannula; IV with D5W at KVO rate; cardiac monitor
    c. Oxygen at 10 L per endotracheal tube; rapid IV infusion of RL; cardiac monitor
    d. Oxygen via nonrebreathing mask; IV; cardiac monitor; immediate transport to hospital

94. Which of the following is *not* a trait of malignant or dangerous PVCs?
    a. Unifocal premature complexes
    b. R on T phenomenon
    c. Greater than six per minute
    d. Runs of ventricular tachycardia

95. All the following are treatments for witnessed ventricular fibrillation, when a defibrillator is available:
  1. Immediate endotracheal intubation
  2. Begin Cardiopulmonary Resuscitation
  3. Defibrillate as recommended by manufacturer
  4. Establish IV access and infuse Normal Saline

The correct sequence for these treatments is:
    a. 2, 3, 1, 4   **c.** 4, 3, 1, 2
    b. 1, 2, 3, 4   **d.** 3, 2, 4, 1

96. Your patient is an 82-year-old woman with a history of coronary artery disease. She is conscious and alert. She is complaining of substernal chest pain, radiating into the left arm. She is diaphoretic and short of breath. Vital signs are: BP = 120/64, pulse = 56 and irregular, respirations = 32, shallow and congested. You connect the cardiac monitor, and it shows ventricular fibrillation. Your immediate action is to:
    a. Begin CPR
    b. Prepare to defibrillate at 200 Joules
    c. Check the monitor leads
    d. Defibrillate at 360 Joules

97. You observe an EKG pattern of "irregular irregularity" on an EKG strip. This strip indicates:
    a. Atrial flutter   **c.** Atrial tachycardia
    b. Atrial fibrillation   **d.** Ventricular pacemaker

98. Because permanent pacemakers are susceptible to damage from strong electrical stimuli, you should never defibrillate a patient who has an implanted pacemaker at a setting higher than 200 Joules.
    a. False   **b.** True

99. A first-degree AV block is a delay in conduction at the level of the AV node rather than an actual block and is not generally considered a dangerous condition.
    a. True   **b.** False

100. Second-degree AV block (Mobitz type II) may be associated with acute myocardial infarction and septal necrosis and is considered to be more serious than Wenckebach (Mobitz type I).
    a. True   **b.** False

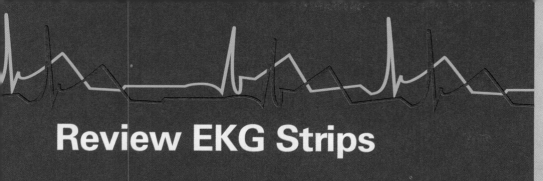

Review EKG Strips

Note:

- Rate and rhythm refer to ventricular rate and rhythm, unless otherwise noted.
- A denotes absent.
- I denotes indistinguishable.

INTRODUCTION

This chapter is included in order to provide review strips that will reinforce your newly acquired knowledge of EKG interpretation. I encourage you to apply the five-step approach to interpret each of the following rhythm strips.

When you have completed this chapter, check your answers with the answers provided in Appendix 2. It should not be assumed that all strips are 6-second strips. You should carefully count the seconds in each strip so that you will reinforce your interpretative skills.

Good luck! Enjoy applying your newly acquired EKG interpretive skills to interpret these review strips.

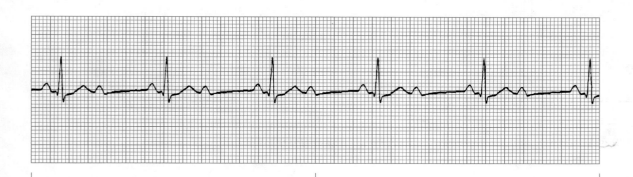

1. Rate: _____ Rhythm: _____

  P wave: _____ PRI: _____

  QRS complex: _____ Interpretation: _____

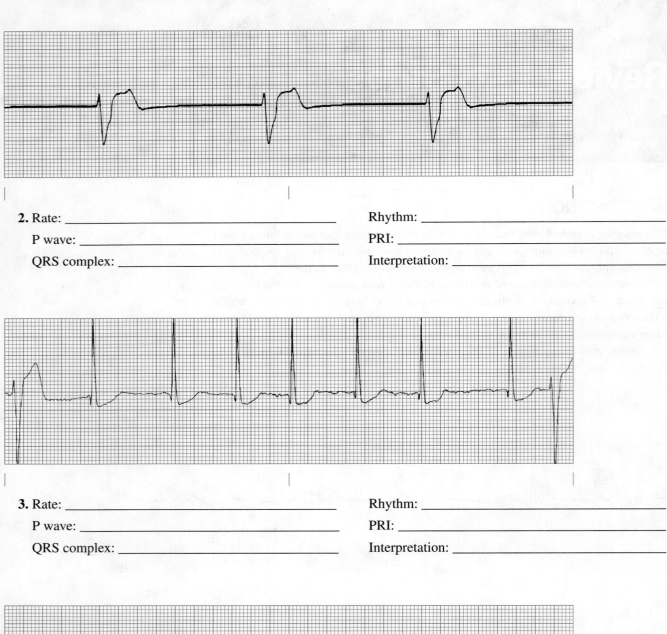

2. Rate: _____   Rhythm: _____

P wave: _____   PRI: _____

QRS complex: _____   Interpretation: _____

3. Rate: _____   Rhythm: _____

P wave: _____   PRI: _____

QRS complex: _____   Interpretation: _____

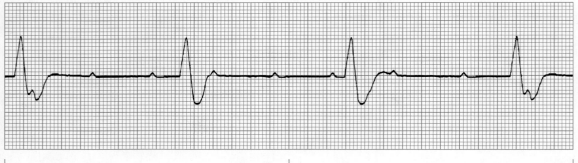

4. Rate: _____   Rhythm: _____

P wave: _____   PRI: _____

QRS complex: _____   Interpretation: _____

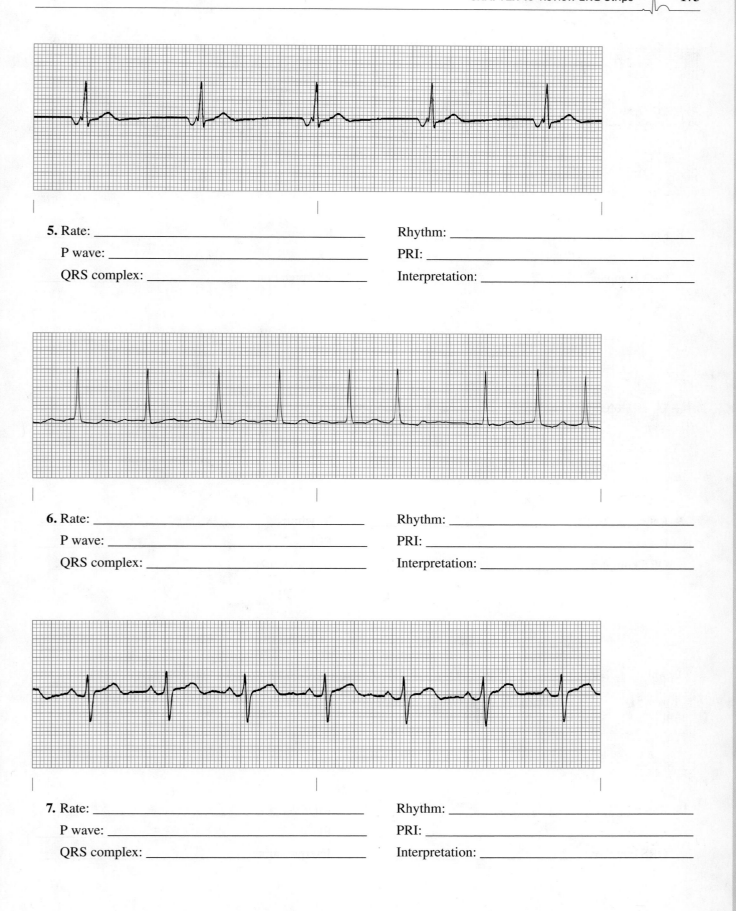

5. Rate: _____   Rhythm: _____

   P wave: _____   PRI: _____

   QRS complex: _____   Interpretation: _____

6. Rate: _____   Rhythm: _____

   P wave: _____   PRI: _____

   QRS complex: _____   Interpretation: _____

7. Rate: _____   Rhythm: _____

   P wave: _____   PRI: _____

   QRS complex: _____   Interpretation: _____

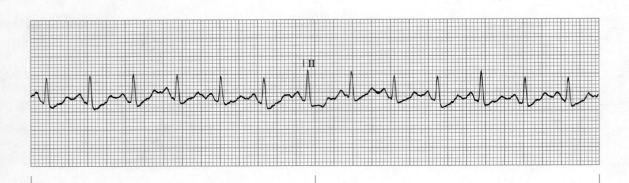

8. Rate: _____   Rhythm: _____

   P wave: _____   PRI: _____

   QRS complex: _____   Interpretation: _____

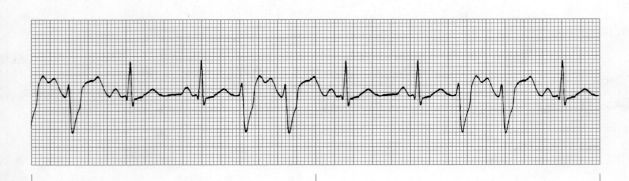

9. Rate: _____   Rhythm: _____

   P wave: _____   PRI: _____

   QRS complex: _____   Interpretation: _____

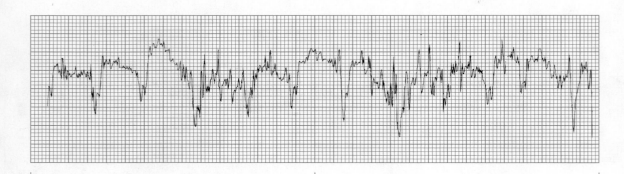

10. Rate: _____   Rhythm: _____

   P wave: _____   PRI: _____

   QRS complex: _____   Interpretation: _____

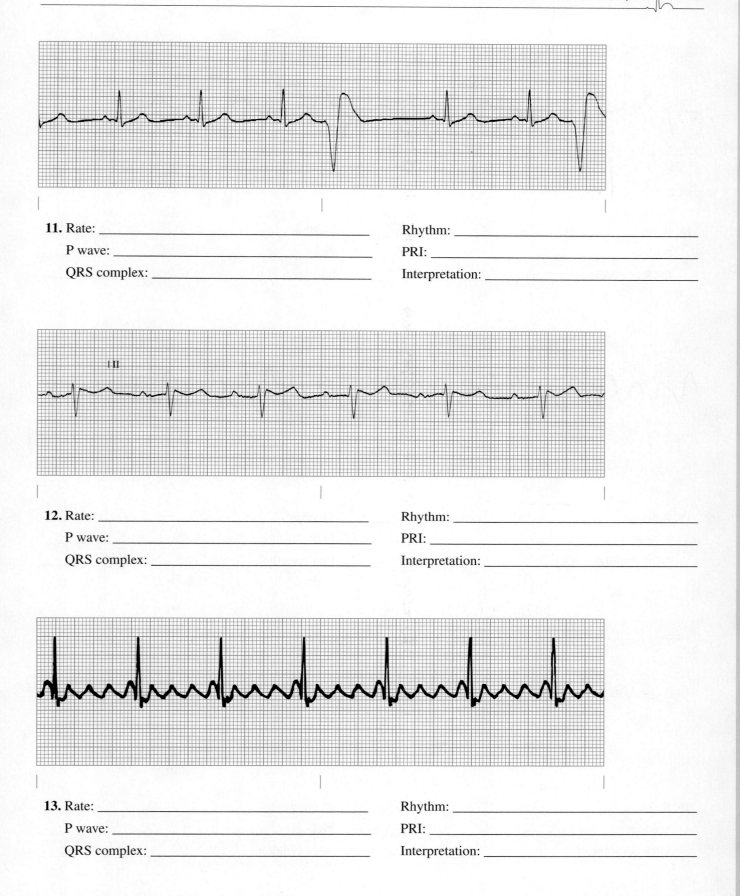

11. Rate: _____   Rhythm: _____

P wave: _____   PRI: _____

QRS complex: _____   Interpretation: _____

12. Rate: _____   Rhythm: _____

P wave: _____   PRI: _____

QRS complex: _____   Interpretation: _____

13. Rate: _____   Rhythm: _____

P wave: _____   PRI: _____

QRS complex: _____   Interpretation: _____

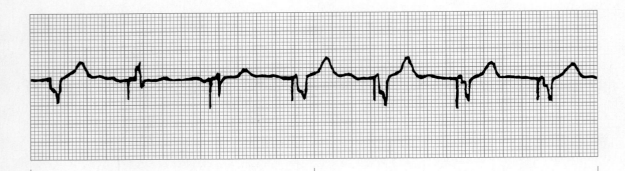

14. Rate: _____ Rhythm: _____

P wave: _____ PRI: _____

QRS complex: _____ Interpretation: _____

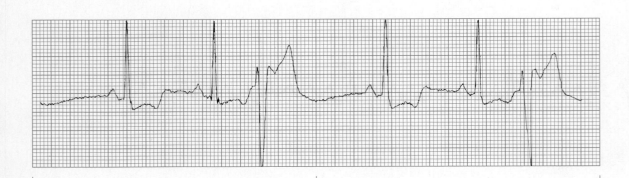

15. Rate: _____ Rhythm: _____

P wave: _____ PRI: _____

QRS complex: _____ Interpretation: _____

16. Rate: _____ Rhythm: _____

P wave: _____ PRI: _____

QRS complex: _____ Interpretation: _____

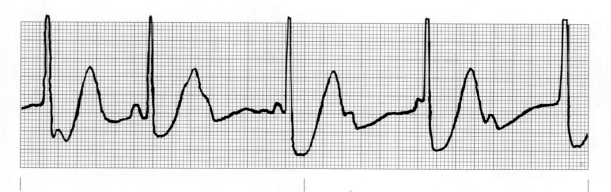

17. Rate: _____   Rhythm: _____

    P wave: _____   PRI: _____

    QRS complex: _____   Interpretation: _____

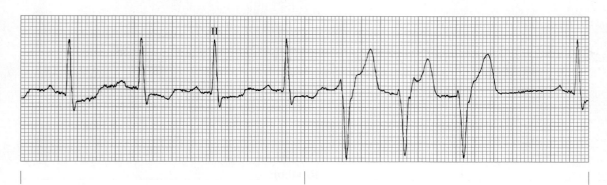

18. Rate: _____   Rhythm: _____

    P wave: _____   PRI: _____

    QRS complex: _____   Interpretation: _____

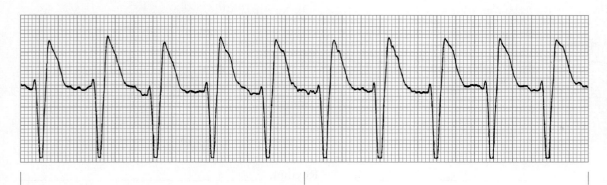

19. Rate: _____   Rhythm: _____

    P wave: _____   PRI: _____

    QRS complex: _____   Interpretation: _____

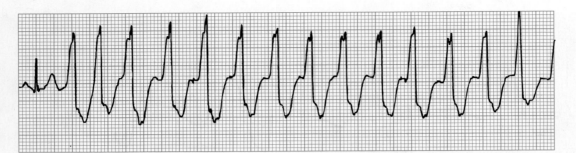

20. Rate: _____   Rhythm: _____

   P wave: _____   PRI: _____

   QRS complex: _____   Interpretation: _____

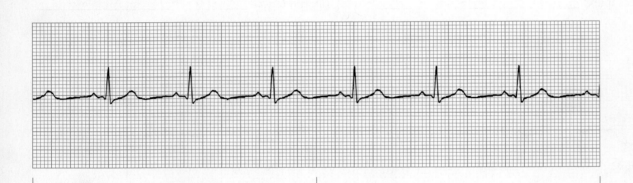

21. Rate: _____   Rhythm: _____

   P wave: _____   PRI: _____

   QRS complex: _____   Interpretation: _____

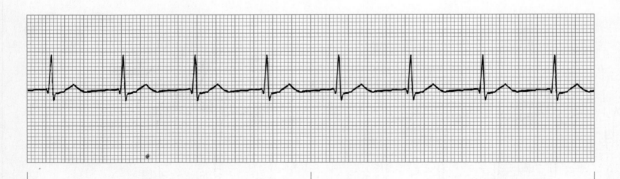

22. Rate: _____   Rhythm: _____

   P wave: _____   PRI: _____

   QRS complex: _____   Interpretation: _____

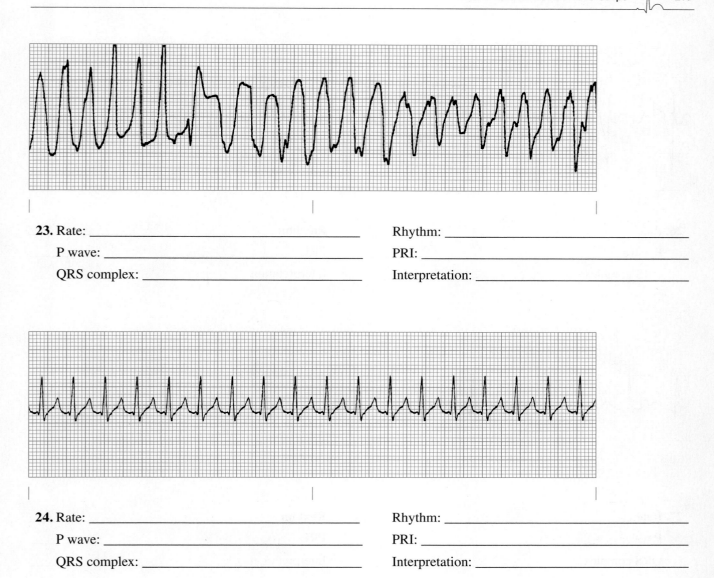

23. Rate: _____ Rhythm: _____

P wave: _____ PRI: _____

QRS complex: _____ Interpretation: _____

24. Rate: _____ Rhythm: _____

P wave: _____ PRI: _____

QRS complex: _____ Interpretation: _____

25. Rate: _____ Rhythm: _____

P wave: _____ PRI: _____

QRS complex: _____ Interpretation: _____

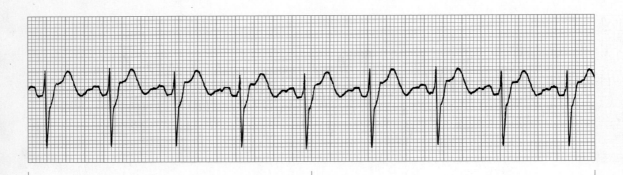

26. Rate: _____ Rhythm: _____

 P wave: _____ PRI: _____

 QRS complex: _____ Interpretation: _____

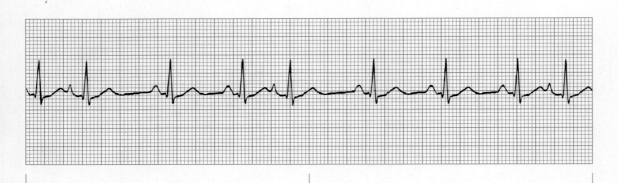

27. Rate: _____ Rhythm: _____

 P wave: _____ PRI: _____

 QRS complex: _____ Interpretation: _____

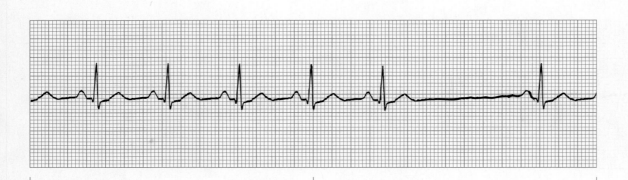

28. Rate: _____ Rhythm: _____

 P wave: _____ PRI: _____

 QRS complex: _____ Interpretation: _____

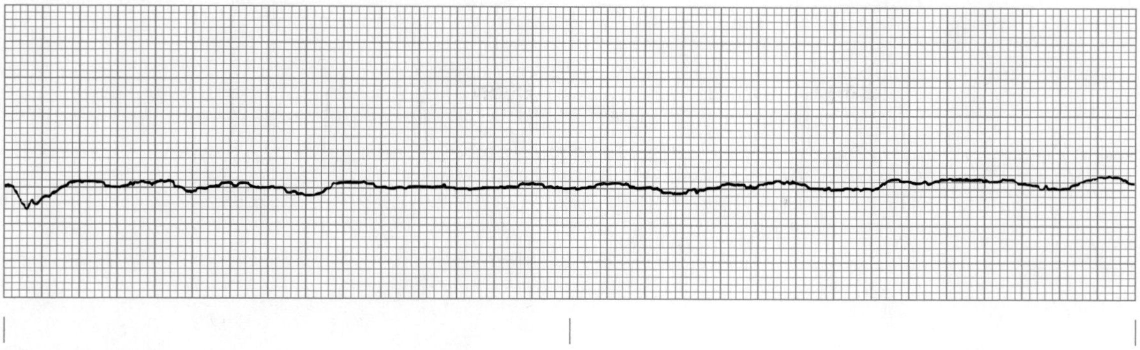

29. Rate: _____   Rhythm: _____

   P wave: _____   PRI: _____

   QRS complex: _____   Interpretation: _____

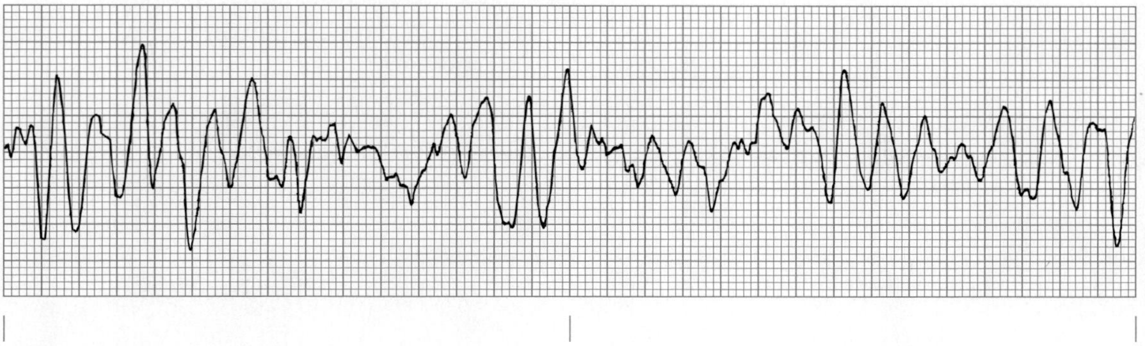

30. Rate: _____   Rhythm: _____

   P wave: _____   PRI: _____

   QRS complex: _____   Interpretation: _____

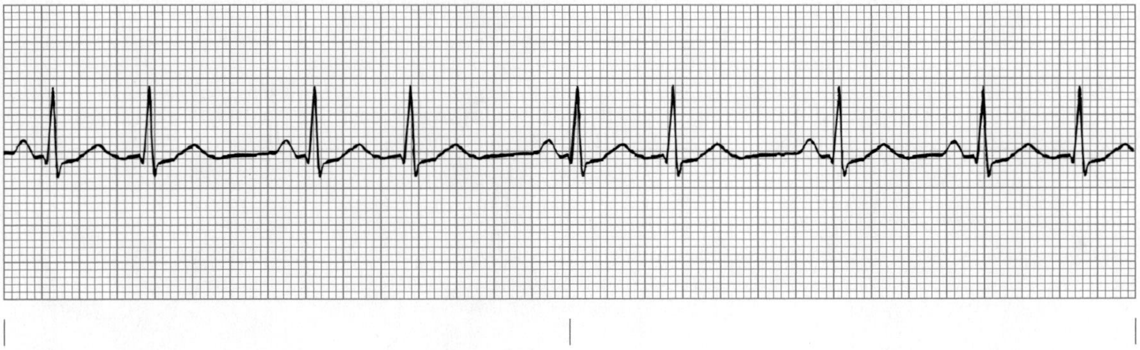

31. Rate: _____   Rhythm: _____

   P wave: _____   PRI: _____

   QRS complex: _____   Interpretation: _____

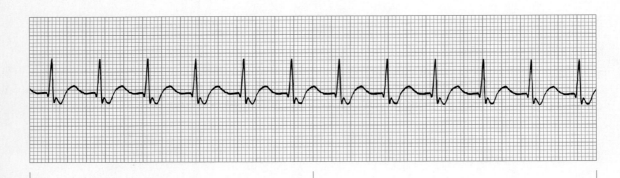

32. Rate: _____ Rhythm: _____

    P wave: _____ PRI: _____

    QRS complex: _____ Interpretation: _____

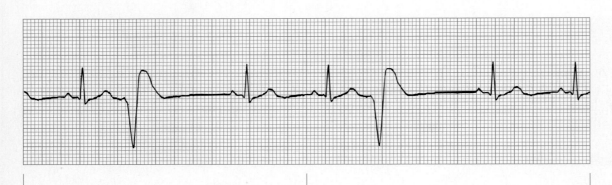

33. Rate: _____ Rhythm: _____

    P wave: _____ PRI: _____

    QRS complex: _____ Interpretation: _____

34. Rate: _____ Rhythm: _____

    P wave: _____ PRI: _____

    QRS complex: _____ Interpretation: _____

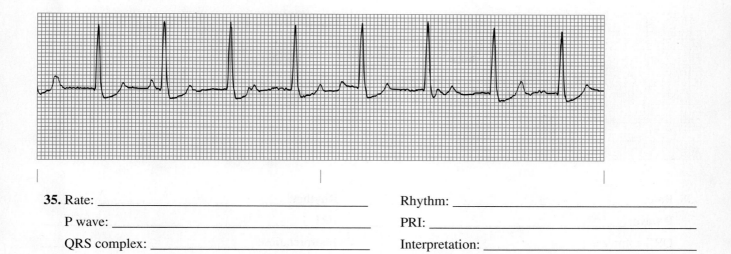

35. Rate: _____ Rhythm: _____

P wave: _____ PRI: _____

QRS complex: _____ Interpretation: _____

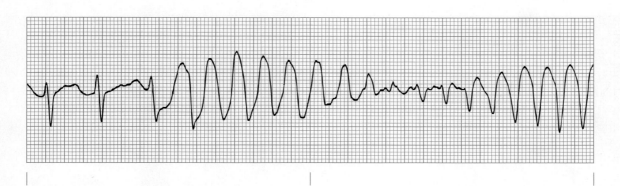

36. Rate: _____ Rhythm: _____

P wave: _____ PRI: _____

QRS complex: _____ Interpretation: _____

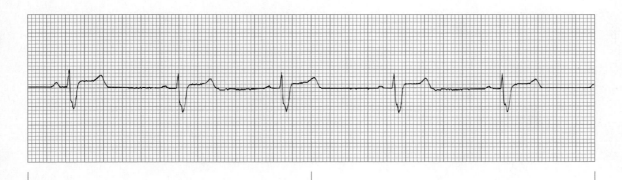

37. Rate: _____ Rhythm: _____

P wave: _____ PRI: _____

QRS complex: _____ Interpretation: _____

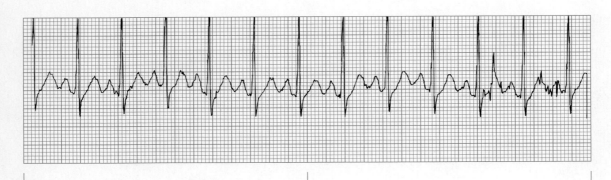

38. Rate: _____ Rhythm: _____

P wave: _____ PRI: _____

QRS complex: _____ Interpretation: _____

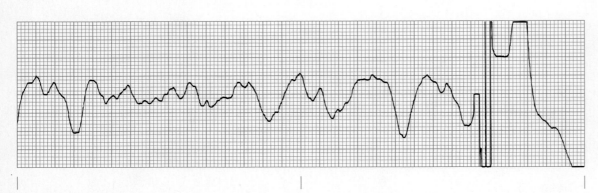

39. Rate: _____ Rhythm: _____

P wave: _____ PRI: _____

QRS complex: _____ Interpretation: _____

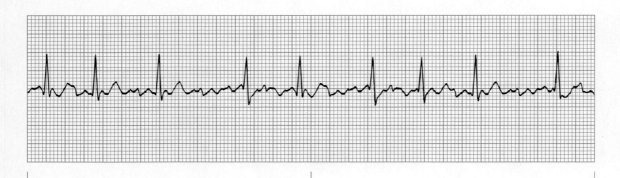

40. Rate: _____ Rhythm: _____

P wave: _____ PRI: _____

QRS complex: _____ Interpretation: _____

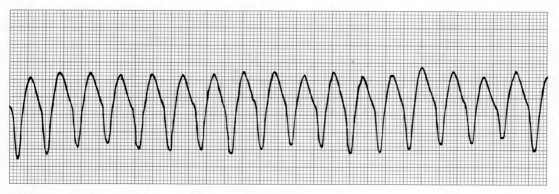

41. Rate: _____   Rhythm: _____

P wave: _____   PRI: _____

QRS complex: _____   Interpretation: _____

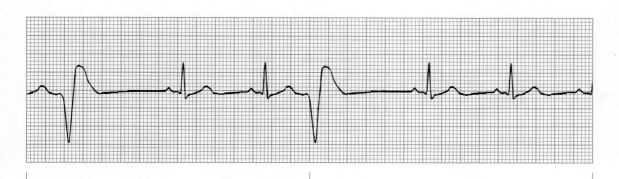

42. Rate: _____   Rhythm: _____

P wave: _____   PRI: _____

QRS complex: _____   Interpretation: _____

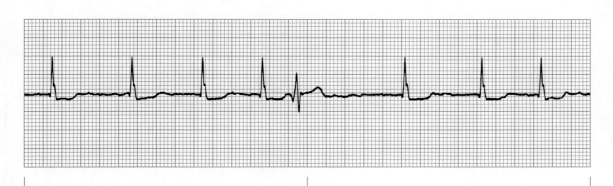

43. Rate: _____   Rhythm: _____

P wave: _____   PRI: _____

QRS complex: _____   Interpretation: _____

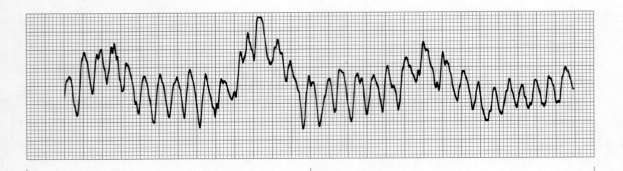

44. Rate: _____   Rhythm: _____

   P wave: _____   PRI: _____

   QRS complex: _____   Interpretation: _____

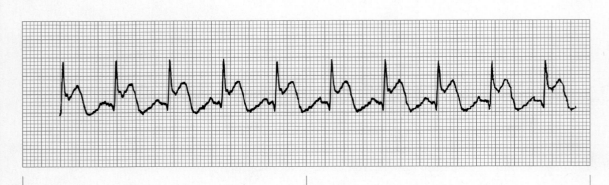

45. Rate: _____   Rhythm: _____

   P wave: _____   PRI: _____

   QRS complex: _____   Interpretation: _____

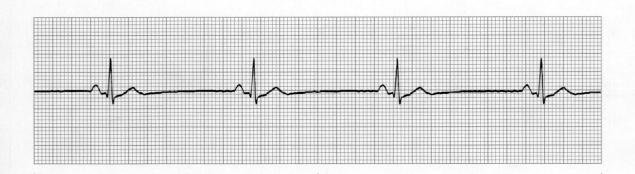

46. Rate: _____   Rhythm: _____

   P wave: _____   PRI: _____

   QRS complex: _____   Interpretation: _____

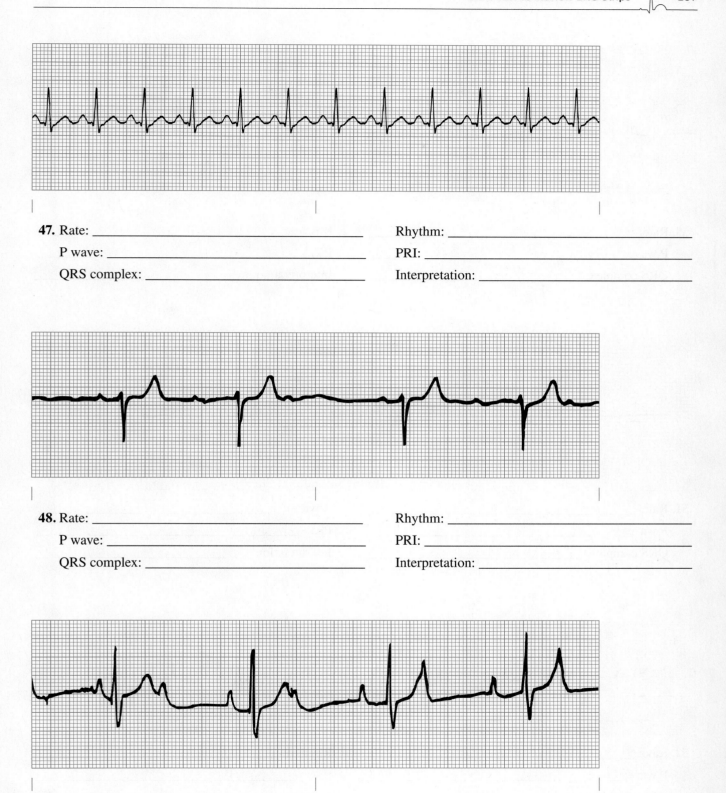

47. Rate: _____   Rhythm: _____

　　　P wave: _____   PRI: _____

　　　QRS complex: _____   Interpretation: _____

48. Rate: _____   Rhythm: _____

　　　P wave: _____   PRI: _____

　　　QRS complex: _____   Interpretation: _____

49. Rate: _____   Rhythm: _____

　　　P wave: _____   PRI: _____

　　　QRS complex: _____   Interpretation: _____

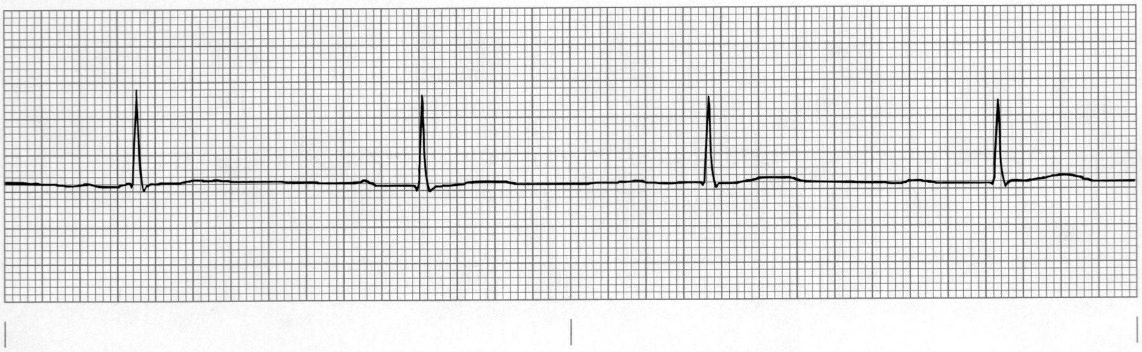

50. Rate: _____   Rhythm: _____

     P wave: _____   PRI: _____

     QRS complex: _____   Interpretation: _____

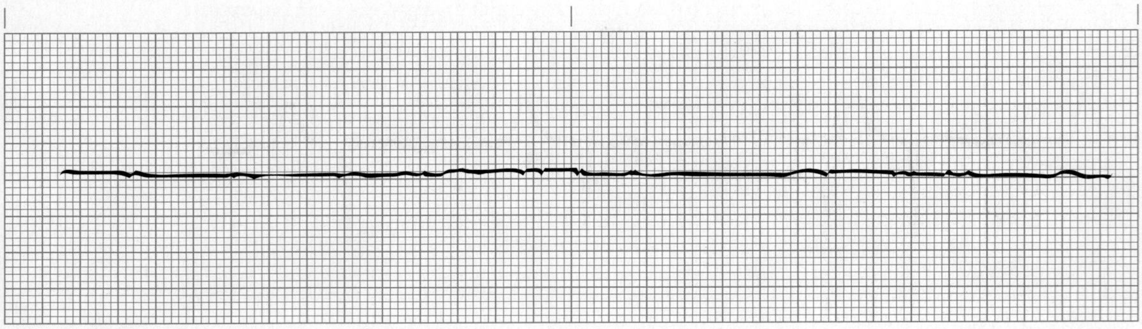

51. Rate: _____   Rhythm: _____

     P wave: _____   PRI: _____

     QRS complex: _____   Interpretation: _____

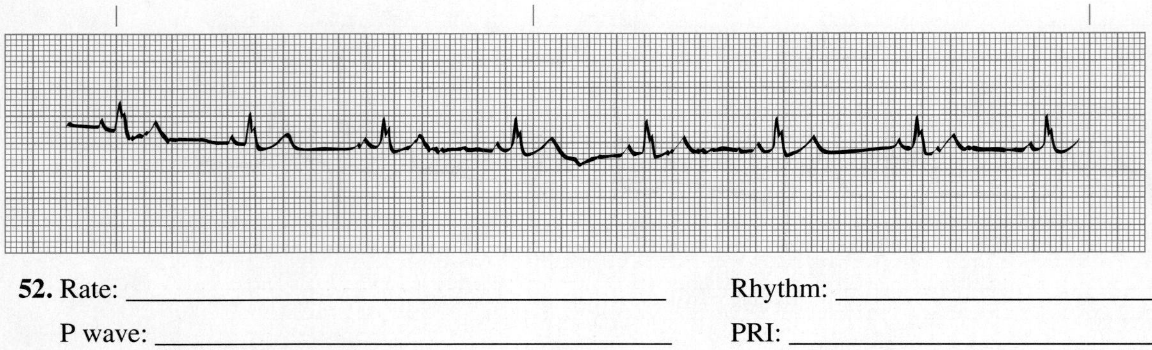

52. Rate: _____   Rhythm: _____

     P wave: _____   PRI: _____

     QRS complex: _____   Interpretation: _____

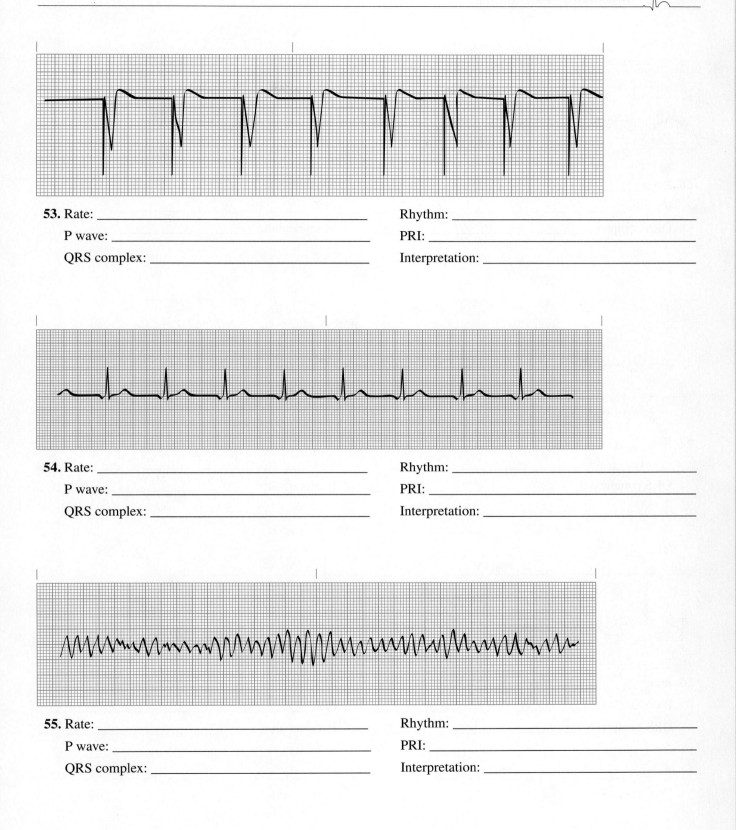

53. Rate: _____   Rhythm: _____

   P wave: _____   PRI: _____

   QRS complex: _____   Interpretation: _____

54. Rate: _____   Rhythm: _____

   P wave: _____   PRI: _____

   QRS complex: _____   Interpretation: _____

55. Rate: _____   Rhythm: _____

   P wave: _____   PRI: _____

   QRS complex: _____   Interpretation: _____

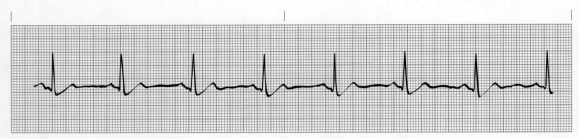

56. Rate: _____   Rhythm: _____

P wave: _____   PRI: _____

QRS complex: _____   Interpretation: _____

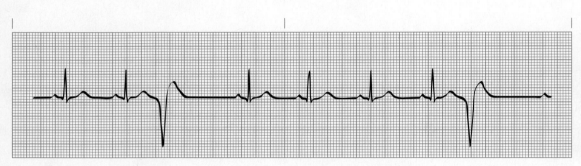

57. Rate: _____   Rhythm: _____

P wave: _____   PRI: _____

QRS complex: _____   Interpretation: _____

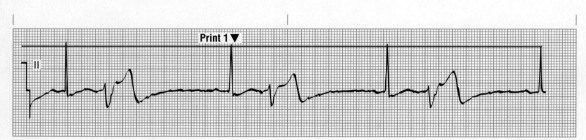

58. Rate: _____   Rhythm: _____

P wave: _____   PRI: _____

QRS complex: _____   Interpretation: _____

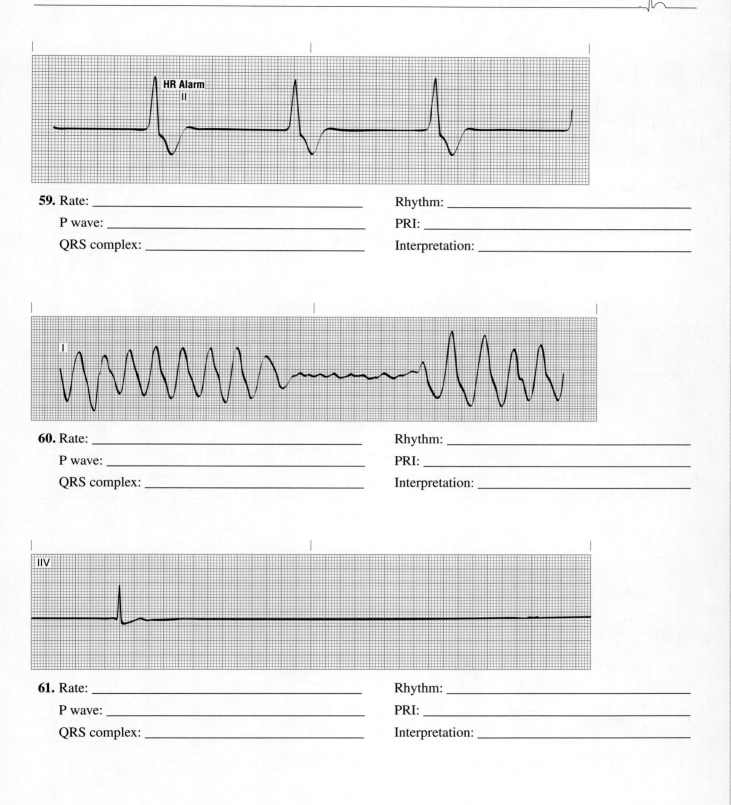

59. Rate: _____ Rhythm: _____

P wave: _____ PRI: _____

QRS complex: _____ Interpretation: _____

60. Rate: _____ Rhythm: _____

P wave: _____ PRI: _____

QRS complex: _____ Interpretation: _____

61. Rate: _____ Rhythm: _____

P wave: _____ PRI: _____

QRS complex: _____ Interpretation: _____

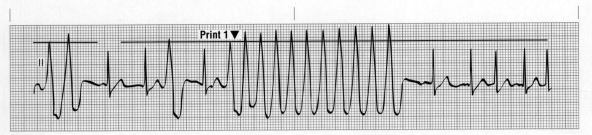

62. Rate: _____   Rhythm: _____

    P wave: _____   PRI: _____

    QRS complex: _____   Interpretation: _____

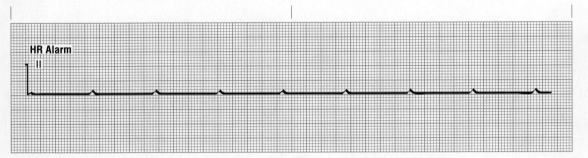

63. Rate: _____   Rhythm: _____

    P wave: _____   PRI: _____

    QRS complex: _____   Interpretation: _____

64. Rate: _____   Rhythm: _____

    P wave: _____   PRI: _____

    QRS complex: _____   Interpretation: _____

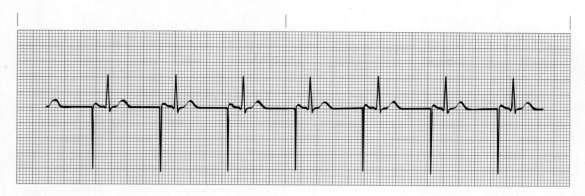

65. Rate: _____   Rhythm: _____

P wave: _____   PRI: _____

QRS complex: _____   Interpretation: _____

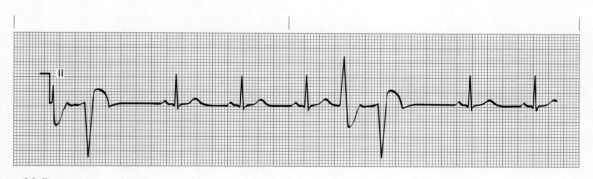

66. Rate: _____   Rhythm: _____

P wave: _____   PRI: _____

QRS complex: _____   Interpretation: _____

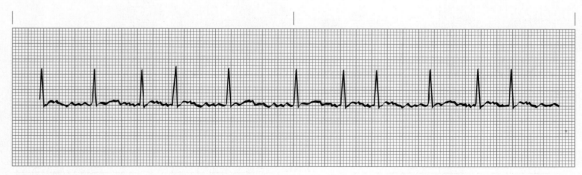

67. Rate: _____   Rhythm: _____

P wave: _____   PRI: _____

QRS complex: _____   Interpretation: _____

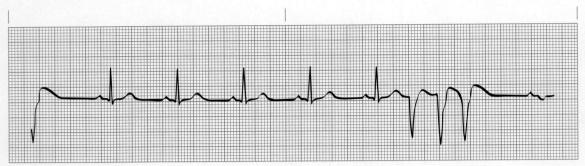

68. Rate: _____   Rhythm: _____

P wave: _____   PRI: _____

QRS complex: _____   Interpretation: _____

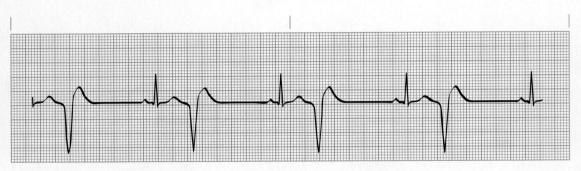

69. Rate: _____   Rhythm: _____

P wave: _____   PRI: _____

QRS complex: _____   Interpretation: _____

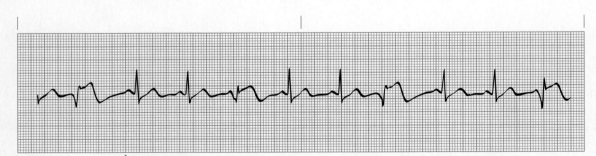

70. Rate: _____   Rhythm: _____

P wave: _____   PRI: _____

QRS complex: _____   Interpretation: _____

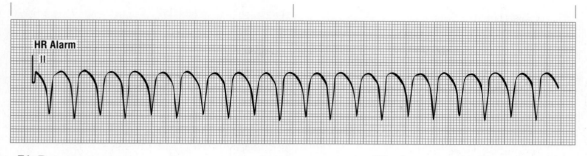

71. Rate: _____ Rhythm: _____

P wave: _____ PRI: _____

QRS complex: _____ Interpretation: _____

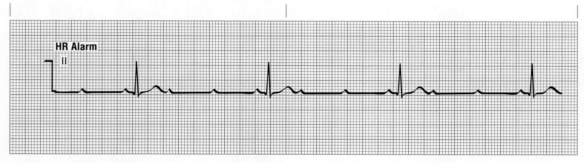

72. Rate: _____ Rhythm: _____

P wave: _____ PRI: _____

QRS complex: _____ Interpretation: _____

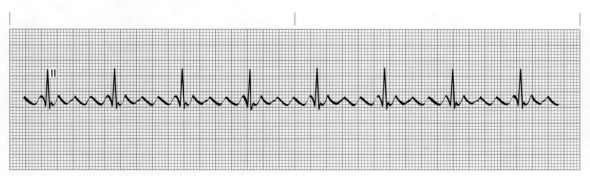

73. Rate: _____ Rhythm: _____

P wave: _____ PRI: _____

QRS complex: _____ Interpretation: _____

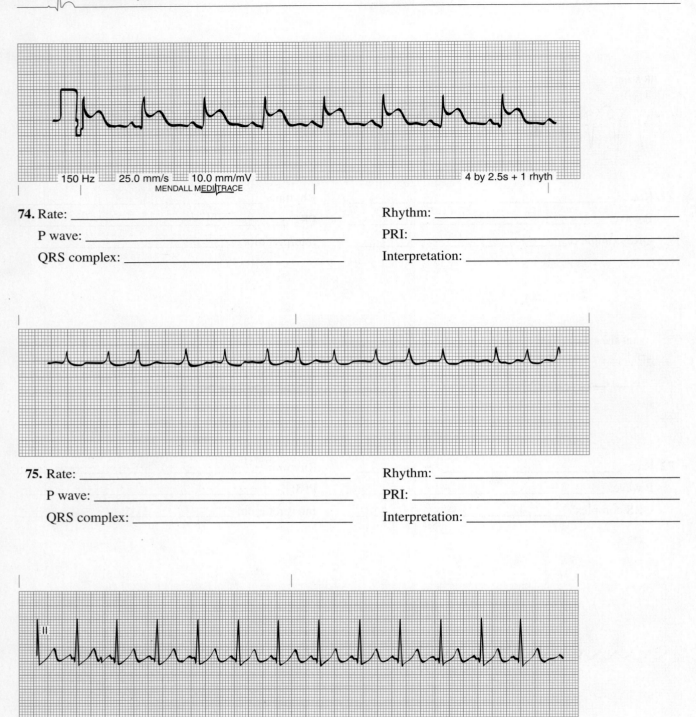

150 Hz   25.0 mm/s   10.0 mm/mV   4 by 2.5s + 1 rhyth
MENDALL MEDITRACE

74. Rate: _____   Rhythm: _____

P wave: _____   PRI: _____

QRS complex: _____   Interpretation: _____

75. Rate: _____   Rhythm: _____

P wave: _____   PRI: _____

QRS complex: _____   Interpretation: _____

II

76. Rate: _____   Rhythm: _____

P wave: _____   PRI: _____

QRS complex: _____   Interpretation: _____

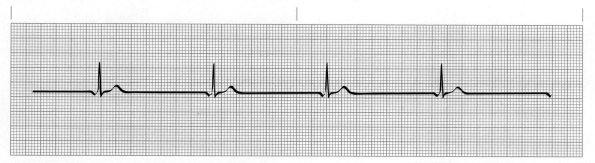

77. Rate: _____   Rhythm: _____

    P wave: _____   PRI: _____

    QRS complex: _____   Interpretation: _____

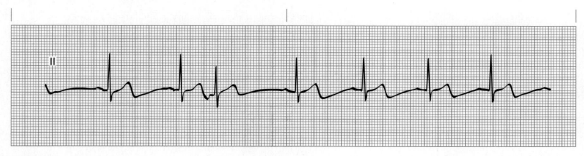

78. Rate: _____   Rhythm: _____

    P wave: _____   PRI: _____

    QRS complex: _____   Interpretation: _____

79. Rate: _____   Rhythm: _____

    P wave: _____   PRI: _____

    QRS complex: _____   Interpretation: _____

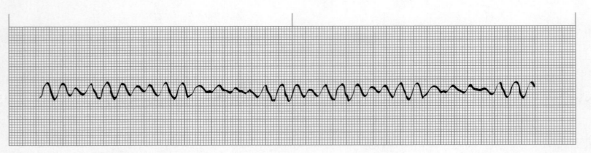

80. Rate: _____ Rhythm: _____

P wave: _____ PRI: _____

QRS complex: _____ Interpretation: _____

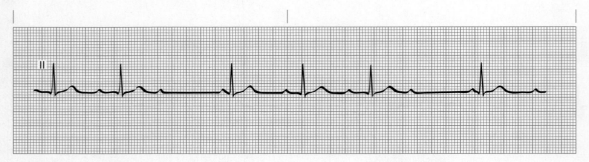

81. Rate: _____ Rhythm: _____

P wave: _____ PRI: _____

QRS complex: _____ Interpretation: _____

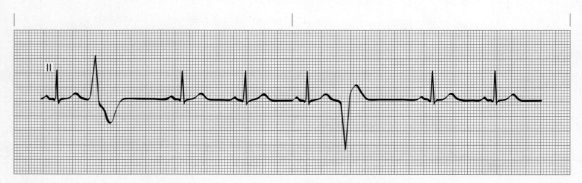

82. Rate: _____ Rhythm: _____

P wave: _____ PRI: _____

QRS complex: _____ Interpretation: _____

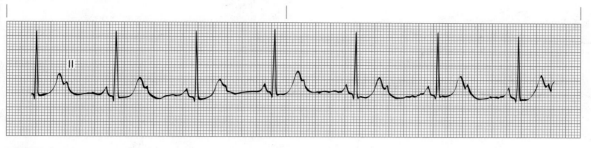

83. Rate: _____   Rhythm: _____

P wave: _____   PRI: _____

QRS complex: _____   Interpretation: _____

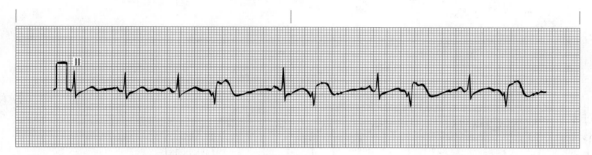

84. Rate: _____   Rhythm: _____

P wave: _____   PRI: _____

QRS complex: _____   Interpretation: _____

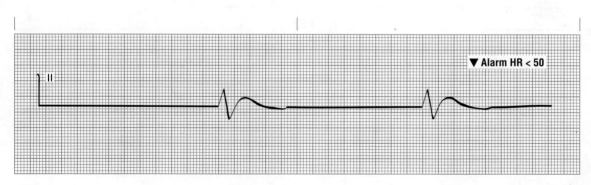

85. Rate: _____   Rhythm: _____

P wave: _____   PRI: _____

QRS complex: _____   Interpretation: _____

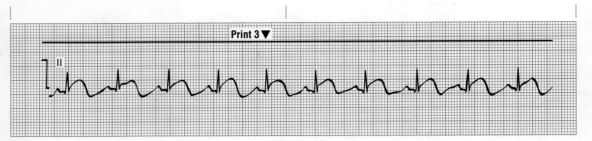

86. Rate: _____ Rhythm: _____

P wave: _____ PRI: _____

QRS complex: _____ Interpretation: _____

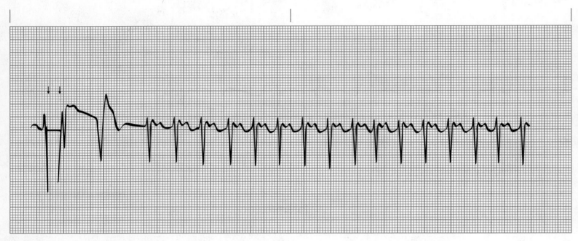

87. Rate: _____ Rhythm: _____

P wave: _____ PRI: _____

QRS complex: _____ Interpretation: _____

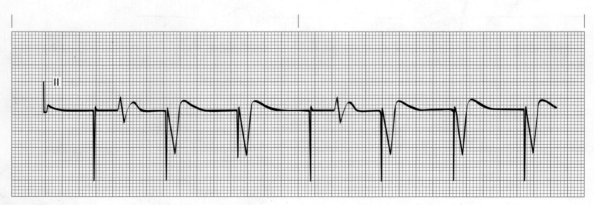

88. Rate: _____ Rhythm: _____

P wave: _____ PRI: _____

QRS complex: _____ Interpretation: _____

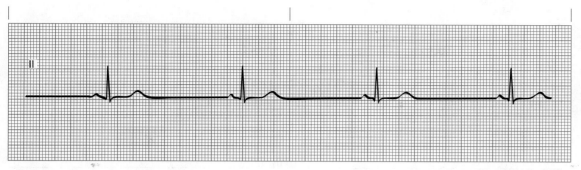

89. Rate: _____   Rhythm: _____

P wave: _____   PRI: _____

QRS complex: _____   Interpretation: _____

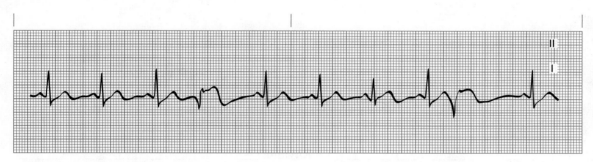

90. Rate: _____   Rhythm: _____

P wave: _____   PRI: _____

QRS complex: _____   Interpretation: _____

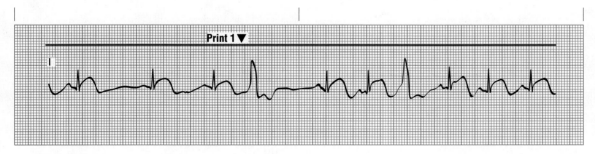

91. Rate: _____   Rhythm: _____

P wave: _____   PRI: _____

QRS complex: _____   Interpretation: _____

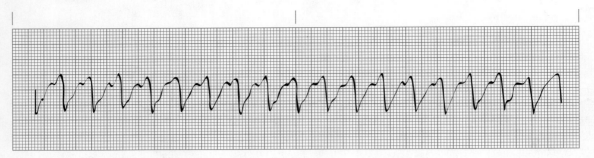

92. Rate: _____   Rhythm: _____

P wave: _____   PRI: _____

QRS complex: _____   Interpretation: _____

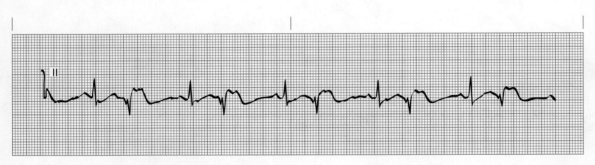

93. Rate: _____   Rhythm: _____

P wave: _____   PRI: _____

QRS complex: _____   Interpretation: _____

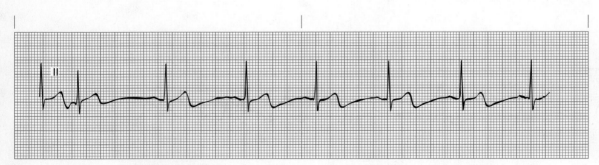

94. Rate: _____   Rhythm: _____

P wave: _____   PRI: _____

QRS complex: _____   Interpretation: _____

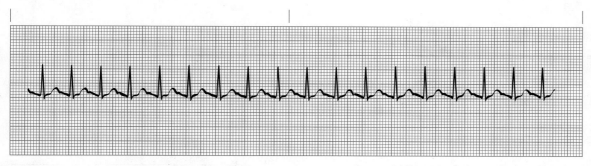

95. Rate: _____ Rhythm: _____

P wave: _____ PRI: _____

QRS complex: _____ Interpretation: _____

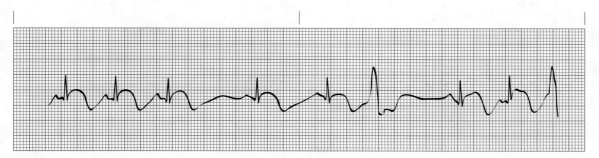

96. Rate: _____ Rhythm: _____

P wave: _____ PRI: _____

QRS complex: _____ Interpretation: _____

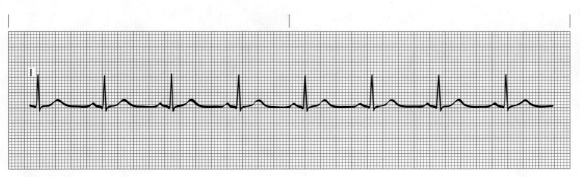

97. Rate: _____ Rhythm: _____

P wave: _____ PRI: _____

QRS complex: _____ Interpretation: _____

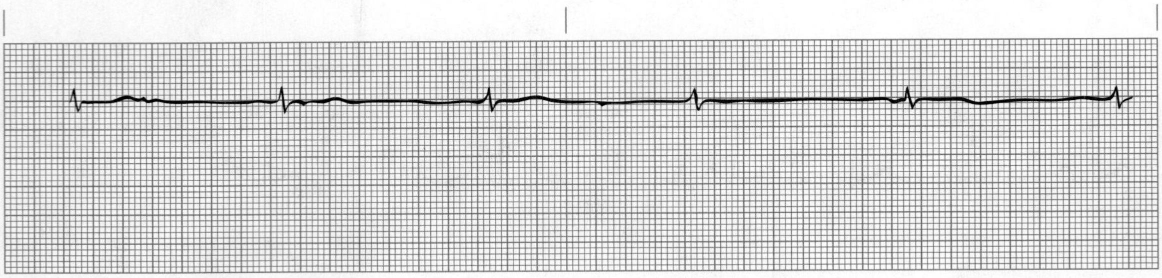

98. Rate: _____ Rhythm: _____

P wave: _____ PRI: _____

QRS complex: _____ Interpretation: _____

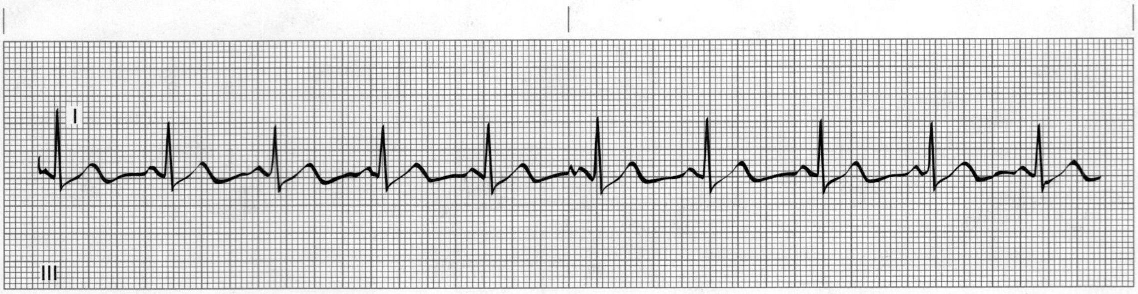

99. Rate: _____ Rhythm: _____

P wave: _____ PRI: _____

QRS complex: _____ Interpretation: _____

25.0 mm/s   10.0 mm/mV   4 by 2.5s   1 rhythm id   V

KENDALL MEDITRACE

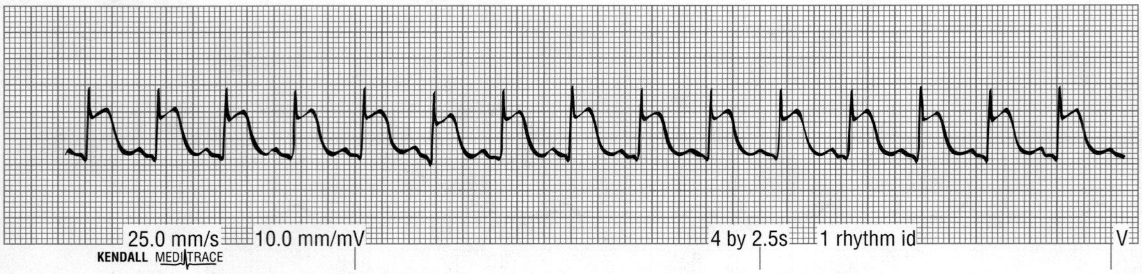

100. Rate: _____ Rhythm: _____

P wave: _____ PRI: _____

QRS complex: _____ Interpretation: _____

Appendix 1

Answers to Review Questions: Chapters 1–14

CHAPTER 1

1. c	**2.** b	**3.** a
4. c	**5.** a	**6.** b
7. d	**8.** c	**9.** b
10. c	**11.** b	**12.** a
13. d	**14.** b	**15.** c

CHAPTER 2

1. b	**2.** b	**3.** b
4. d	**5.** a	**6.** c
7. b	**8.** d	**9.** a
10. b	**11.** c	**12.** d
13. c	**14.** d	**15.** a

CHAPTER 3

1. c	**2.** a	**3.** a
4. d	**5.** a	**6.** d
7. a	**8.** a	**9.** a
10. a	**11.** c	**12.** a
13. b	**14.** c	**15.** d

CHAPTER 4

1. a	**2.** a	**3.** d
4. c	**5.** c	**6.** b
7. c	**8.** c	**9.** b
10. c	**11.** b	**12.** a
13. b	**14.** c	**15.** c

CHAPTER 5

1. b	**2.** c	**3.** d
4. b	**5.** d	**6.** b
7. a	**8.** a	**9.** d
10. b	**11.** a	**12.** a
13. c	**14.** a	**15.** a

CHAPTER 6

1. b	**2.** d	**3.** a
4. c	**5.** d	**6.** b
7. a	**8.** d	**9.** b
10. a	**11.** a	**12.** d
13. a	**14.** b	**15.** a

CHAPTER 7

1. c	**2.** b	**3.** a
4. d	**5.** d	**6.** a
7. b	**8.** a	**9.** b
10. d	**11.** a	**12.** a
13. a	**14.** a	**15.** a

Chapter 7 (Review Strips)

1. Rate: 75
   Rhythm: Regular
   P wave: Present and upright
   PRI: 0.18
   QRS: 0.06
   Interpretation: Normal sinus rhythm
2. Rate: 110
   Rhythm: Regular
   P wave: Present and upright
   PRI: 0.16
   QRS: 0.06
   Interpretation: Sinus tachycardia
3. Rate: 50
   Rhythm: Regular
   P wave: Present and upright
   PRI: 0.14
   QRS: 0.08
   Interpretation: Sinus bradycardia
4. Rate: 70
   Rhythm: Irregular
   P wave: Present and upright
   PRI: 0.16
   QRS: 0.08
   Interpretation: Sinus dysrhythmia
5. Rate: 40
   Rhythm: Irregular
   P wave: Present and upright
   PRI: 0.20
   QRS: 0.06
   Interpretation: Sinus brady with sinus arrest

6. Rate: 70
   Rhythm: Irregular
   P wave: Present and upright
   PRI: 0.16
   QRS: 0.08
   Interpretation: Sinus dysrhythmia

7. Rate: 136
   Rhythm: Regular
   P wave: Present and upright
   PRI: 0.18
   QRS: 0.06
   Interpretation: Sinus tachycardia

8. Rate: 80
   Rhythm: Irregular
   P wave: Present and upright
   PRI: 0.16
   QRS: 0.04
   Interpretation: Sinus dysrhythmia

9. Rate: 50
   Rhythm: Regular
   P wave: Present and upright
   PRI: 0.14
   QRS: 0.06
   Interpretation: Sinus bradycardia

10. Rate: 60
    Rhythm: Irregular
    P wave: Present and upright
    PRI: 0.16
    QRS: 0.08
    Interpretation: Sinus arrest rhythm

CHAPTER 8

1. a	**2.** a	**3.** b
4. d	**5.** c	**6.** d
7. a	**8.** a	**9.** a
10. d	**11.** a	**12.** b
13. c	**14.** b	**15.** d

Chapter 8 (Review Strips)

1. Rate: 50
   Rhythm: Regular
   P wave: Present and upright
   PRI: Varies with varying morphology
   QRS: 0.04
   Interpretation: Wandering atrial pacemaker

2. Rate: 80
   Rhythm: Regular
   P wave: Flutter waves
   PRI: Indistinguishable (I)
   QRS: 0.06
   Interpretation: Atrial flutter—4:1 ratio

3. Rate: 60
   Rhythm: Irregularly irregular
   P wave: f waves
   PRI: I
   QRS: 0.08
   Interpretation: Atrial fibrillation

4. Rate: 70
   Rhythm: Irregular
   P wave: Present and upright
   PRI: 0.16
   QRS: 0.06
   Interpretation: Sinus rhythm with PACs

5. Rate: 210
   Rhythm: Regular
   P wave: I
   PRI: I
   QRS: 0.06
   Interpretation: Supraventricular tachycardia

6. Rate: 50
   Rhythm: Irregularly irregular
   P wave: f
   PRI: I
   QRS: 0.06
   Interpretation: Atrial fibrillation

7. Rate: 80
   Rhythm: Irregular
   P wave: Present and upright
   PRI: 0.14
   QRS: 0.10
   Interpretation: Sinus rhythm with a PAC

8. Rate: 90
   Rhythm: Irregular
   P wave: Flutter waves
   PRI: I
   QRS: 0.06
   Interpretation: Atrial flutter: variable ventricular response

9. Rate: 190
   Rhythm: Regular
   P wave: I
   PRI: I
   QRS: 0.08
   Interpretation: Supraventricular tachycardia

10. Rate: 50
    Rhythm: Regular
    P wave: Varying morphology
    PRI: Variable
    QRS: 0.06
    Interpretation: Wandering atrial pacemaker

CHAPTER 9

1. a	**2.** d	**3.** c
4. d	**5.** c	**6.** a
7. c	**8.** c	**9.** b
10. d	**11.** a	**12.** d
13. a	**14.** a	**15.** a

Chapter 9 (Review Strips)

1. Rate: 70
   Rhythm: Regular
   P wave: Present and inverted
   PRI: 0.10
   QRS: 0.06
   Interpretation: Accelerated junctional rhythm

2. Rate: 30
   Rhythm: Regular
   P wave: Absent (A)
   PRI: A
   QRS: 0.06
   Interpretation: Junctional rhythm

3. Rate: 70
   Rhythm: Irregular
   P wave: Present and upright
   PRI: 0.14 except for ectopic beat
   QRS: 0/06
   Interpretation: Sinus rhythm with PJCs

4. Rate: 120
   Rhythm: Regular
   P wave: A
   PRI: A
   QRS: 0.08
   Interpretation: Junctional tachycardia

5. Rate: 70
   Rhythm: Irregular
   P wave: Present and upright
   PRI: 0.16 except for ectopic beats
   QRS: 0.08
   Interpretation: Sinus rhythm with PJCs (bigeminy)

6. Rate: 70
   Rhythm: Regular
   P wave: A
   PRI: A
   QRS: 0.06
   Interpretation: Accelerated junctional rhythm

7. Rate: 40
   Rhythm: Regular
   P wave: Inverted, follow QRS
   PRI: A
   QRS: 0.08
   Interpretation: Junctional rhythm

8. Rate: 120
   Rhythm: Regular
   P wave: A
   PRI: A
   QRS: 0.10
   Interpretation: Junctional tachycardia

CHAPTER 10

1. c	**2.** a	**3.** d
4. c	**5.** b	**6.** b
7. a	**8.** b	**9.** a
10. a	**11.** a	**12.** c
13. a	**14.** c	**15.** d

Chapter 10 (Review Strips)

1. Rate: I
   Rhythm: I
   P wave: A
   PRI: A
   QRS: A
   Interpretation: Coarse ventricular fibrillation

2. Rate: I
   Rhythm: I
   P wave: A
   PRI: A
   QRS: A
   Interpretation: Fine ventricular fibrillation

3. Rate: A
   Rhythm: A
   P wave: A
   PRI: A
   QRS: A
   Interpretation: Asystole

4. Rate: Atrial rate: 40
   Rhythm: Atrial rhythm: regular
   P wave: Present and upright
   PRI: A
   QRS: A
   Interpretation: Ventricular standstill

5. Rate: 140
   Rhythm: Regular
   P wave: A

6. Rate: 110
   Rhythm: Irregular
   P wave: Present and upright

7. Rate: 120
   Rhythm: Irregular
   P wave: Present upright except for ectopic beats

8. Rate: 80
   Rhythm: Irregular
   P wave: Present and upright except for ectopic beats

9. Rate: 70
   Rhythm: Irregular
   P wave: Present and upright except for ectopic beats

10. Rate: I
    Rhythm: I
    P wave: A

11. Rate: 190
    Rhythm: Regular
    P wave: A

12. Rate: 70
    Rhythm: Irregular
    P wave: Present and upright except for ectopic beats

13. Rate: 80
    Rhythm: Irregular
    P wave: Present and upright except for ectopic beats

14. Rate: 40
    Rhythm: Regular
    P wave: A

PRI: A
QRS: 0.28
Interpretation: Ventricular tachycardia

PRI: 0.16
QRS: 0.06
Interpretation: Sinus rhythm with quadrigeminy

PRI: 0.16
QRS: 0.06
Interpretation: Sinus rhythm with couplet PVCs

PRI: 0.16
QRS: 0.04
Interpretation: Sinus rhythm with multifocal PVCs

PRI: 0.20
QRS: 0.08
Interpretation: Sinus rhythm with unifocal PVCs, Trigeminy

PRI: A
QRS: A
Interpretation: Torsades de pointes

PRI: A
QRS: 0.16
Interpretation: Ventricular tachycardia

PRI: 0.18
QRS: 0.08
Interpretation: Sinus rhythm with unifocal PVCs

PRI: 0.16
QRS: 0.08
Interpretation: Sinus rhythm with unifocal PVCs (bigeminy)

PRI: A
QRS: 0.16
Interpretation: Idioventricular rhythm

CHAPTER 11

1. c	**2.** d	**3.** a
4. a	**5.** a	**6.** d
7. a	**8.** b	**9.** c
10. c	**11.** a	**12.** a
13. a	**14.** a	**15.** a

Chapter 11 (Review Strips)

1. Rate: 60
   Rhythm: Regular
   P wave: Present and upright

2. Rate: 70
   Rhythm: Regular
   P wave: Present and upright

3. Rate: 60
   Rhythm: Regular
   P wave: Present and upright

4. Rate: 70
   Rhythm: Irregular
   P wave: Present and upright

PRI: Varies
QRS: 0.04
Interpretation: Third-degree heart block

PRI: 0.22
QRS: 0.06
Interpretation: First-degree heart block

PRI: Varies
QRS: 0.04
Interpretation: Third-degree heart block

PRI: Progressively prolonging until QRS is dropped
QRS: 0.08
Interpretation: Second-degree heart block, Mobitz type I; Wenckebach

5. Rate: 60
   Rhythm: Regular
   P wave: Present and upright
6. Rate: 20
   Rhythm: Regular
   P wave: Present and upright
7. Rate: 40
   Rhythm: Regular
   P wave: Present and upright
8. Rate: 60
   Rhythm: Irregular
   P wave: Present and upright

PRI: 0.28
QRS: 0.08
Interpretation: First-degree heart block
PRI: Variable
QRS: 0.12
Interpretation: Third-degree heart block
PRI: 0.24
QRS: 0.12
Interpretation: Second-degree block, type II, 2:1 conduction
PRI: Progressively prolonging, until QRS is dropped
QRS: 0.08
Interpretation: Second-degree heart block, Mobitz type I; Wenckebach

CHAPTER 12

1. a	**2.** b	**3.** b
4. c	**5.** b	**6.** a
7. a	**8.** a	**9.** a
10. d	**11.** a	**12.** a
13. a	**14.** a	**15.** a

Chapter 12 (Review Strips)

1. Rate: 40
   Rhythm: Regular
   P wave: Varies

2. Rate: 80
   Rhythm: Regular
   P wave: Generated by pacer
3. Rate: 80
   Rhythm: Irregular
   P wave: Present and upright
4. Rate: 70
   Rhythm: Regular
   P wave: A
5. Rate: 90
   Rhythm: Regular
   P wave: A
6. Rate: 50
   Rhythm: Irregular
   P wave: Present and upright

7. Rate: 70
   Rhythm: Regular
   P wave: A
8. Rate: 80
   Rhythm: Irregular
   P wave: A

PRI: Varies
QRS: 0.12
Interpretation: Malfunctioning pacemaker and third-degree block
PRI: 0.14
QRS: 0.16
Interpretation: Sequential AV pacemaker rhythm
PRI: 0.16 in normal complexes
QRS: 0.04
Interpretation: Sinus rhythm with ventricular demand pacer
PRI: A
QRS: 0.14
Interpretation: Ventricular pacemaker rhythm
PRI: A
QRS: 0.14
Interpretation: Ventricular pacemaker rhythm
PRI: 0.24
QRS: 0.08
Interpretation: Malfunctioning pacemaker rhythm; first-degree heart block
PRI: A
QRS: 0.12
Interpretation: Ventricular pacemaker rhythm
PRI: A
QRS: 0.12
Interpretation: Malfunctioning pacemaker rhythm

CHAPTER 13

1. d	**2.** a	**3.** b
4. d	**5.** c	**6.** d
7. b	**8.** b	**9.** d
10. d	**11.** a	**12.** b
13. d	**14.** d	**15.** c
16. c	**17.** b	**18.** a
19. c	**20.** a	

CHAPTER 14

1. a	**2.** c	**3.** b
4. a	**5.** c	**6.** c
7. d	**8.** c	**9.** a
10. b	**11.** d	**12.** c
13. a	**14.** a	**15.** c
16. d	**17.** a	**18.** d
19. d	**20.** c	**21.** c
22. d	**23.** b	**24.** a
25. c	**26.** d	**27.** a
28. d	**29.** d	**30.** d
31. d	**32.** b	**33.** c
34. a	**35.** d	**36.** a
37. d	**38.** a	**39.** a
40. a	**41.** c	**42.** b
43. c	**44.** c	**45.** c
46. a	**47.** a	**48.** b
49. c	**50.** d	**51.** c
52. c	**53.** d	**54.** d
55. b	**56.** c	**57.** b
58. c	**59.** a	**60.** a
61. b	**62.** a	**63.** a
64. a	**65.** c	**66.** b
67. d	**68.** a	**69.** d
70. a	**71.** b	**72.** a
73. b	**74.** a	**75.** a
76. b	**77.** a	**78.** c
79. a	**80.** d	**81.** c
82. d	**83.** a	**84.** d
85. d	**86.** a	**87.** a
88. d	**89.** d	**90.** b
91. b	**92.** b	**93.** d
94. a	**95.** d	**96.** c
97. b	**98.** a	**99.** a
100. a		

Answers to Review Strips: Chapter 15

CHAPTER 15

1. Rate: 60
   Rhythm: Regular
   P wave: 2 per QRS complex
   PRI: 0.16 seconds
   QRS: 0.04 seconds
   Interpretation: Second-degree heart block, Mobitz type II, 2:1 block

2. Rate: 30
   Rhythm: Regular
   P wave: A
   PRI: A
   QRS: 0.14 seconds
   Interpretation: Idioventricular rhythm

3. Rate: 90
   Rhythm: Irregular
   P wave: A
   PRI: A
   QRS: 0.06 seconds
   Interpretation: Atrial fibrillation with unifocal PVCs

4. Rate: Ventricular—40; atrial—80
   Rhythm: Regular
   P wave: Present and upright
   PRI: Variable
   QRS: 0.10 seconds
   Interpretation: Third-degree (complete) heart block

5. Rate: 50
   Rhythm: Regular
   P wave: Inverted
   PRI: 0.08 seconds
   QRS: 0.04 seconds
   Interpretation: Junctional escape rhythm

6. Rate: 90
   Rhythm: Irregular
   P wave: A
   PRI: A
   QRS: 0.04
   Interpretation: Atrial fibrillation

7. Rate: 70
   Rhythm: Regular
   P wave: Present and upright
   PRI: 0.16 seconds
   QRS: 0.08 seconds
   Interpretation: Normal sinus rhythm (NSR)

8. Rate: 130
    Rhythm: Regular
    P wave: Present and upright
    PRI: 0.12 seconds
    QRS: 0.04 seconds
    Interpretation: Sinus tachycardia

9. Rate: 110
    Rhythm: Irregular (due to premature complexes)
    P wave: Present and upright
    PRI: 0.16 seconds
    QRS: 0.04 seconds (for normally conducted beats)
    Interpretation: Sinus rhythm with couplet PVCs

10. Rate: I
    Rhythm: I
    P wave: I
    PRI: I
    QRS: I
    Interpretation: Artifact

11. Rate: 70
    Rhythm: Irregular
    P wave: Present (for sinus complexes)
    PRI: 0.16 seconds
    QRS: 0.06 seconds (sinus complexes); 0.14 seconds (PVCs)
    Interpretation: Sinus rhythm; unifocal premature ventricular complexes

12. Rate: 60
    Rhythm: Regular
    P wave: Present and upright
    PRI: 0.28 seconds
    QRS: 0.04 seconds
    Interpretation: Sinus rhythm with first-degree heart block

13. Rate: 70
    Rhythm: Regular
    P wave: I (flutter waves)
    PRI: I
    QRS: 0.04 seconds
    Interpretation: Atrial flutter (4:1 ratio)

14. Rate: 70
    Rhythm: Paced rhythm
    P wave: A
    PRI: I
    QRS: 0.10 seconds
    Interpretation: Ventricular pacemaker

15. Rate: I
    Rhythm: I
    P wave: I
    PRI: I
    QRS: I
    Interpretation: Coarse ventricular fibrillation

16. Rate: 60
    Rhythm: Irregular (due to premature complexes)
    P wave: Present and upright (for sinus beats)
    PRI: 0.20 seconds
    QRS: 0.06 seconds
    Interpretation: Sinus rhythm with ventricular trigeminy

17. Rate: 50
    Rhythm: Atrial—regular; ventricular—regular (after first QRS, which
                     is a PVC)
    P wave: Present and upright
    PRI: Variable
    QRS: 0.12 seconds
    Interpretation: Third-degree heart block (complete heart block)

18. Rate: 80
    Rhythm: Irregular (due to premature complexes)
    P wave: Present and upright (for sinus beats)
    PRI: 0.20 seconds
    QRS: 0.08 seconds (sinus beats)
    Interpretation: Sinus rhythm, with short run of ventricular tachycardia

19. Rate: 100
    Rhythm: Regular
    P wave: A
    PRI: I
    QRS: 0.12 seconds
    Interpretation: Accelerated idioventricular rhythm

20. Rate: 150
    Rhythm: Irregular
    P wave: Present and upright in first
                     complex only; otherwise absent
    PRI: 0.12 seconds in first complex only; otherwise absent
    QRS: 0.06 seconds in first complex only; in other complexes, greater than 0.12 seconds
    Interpretation: Ventricular tachycardia

21. Rate: 60
    Rhythm: Atrial—regular; ventricular—regular
    P wave: Present and upright
    PRI: 0.16 seconds
    QRS: 0.04 seconds
    Interpretation: Normal sinus rhythm

22. Rate: 80
    Rhythm: Regular
    P wave: A
    PRI: I
    QRS: 0.04 seconds
    Interpretation: Accelerated junctional rhythm

23. Rate: 220
    Rhythm: Irregular
    P wave: I
    PRI: I
    QRS: Variable (0.12–0.24 seconds)
    Interpretation: Torsades de pointes

24. Rate: 180
    Rhythm: Regular
    P wave: Present and upright
    PRI: 0.04 seconds
    QRS: 0.04 seconds
    Interpretation: Supraventricular tachycardia

25. Rate: 80
    Rhythm: Irregular (due to premature complex)
    P wave: Present and upright (for sinus beats)
    PRI: 0.20 seconds
    QRS: 0.04 seconds
    Interpretation: Sinus rhythm with PVCs (premature ventricular complexes)

26. Rate: 90
    Rhythm: Regular
    P wave: Present and upright
    PRI: 0.16 seconds
    QRS: 0.08 seconds
    Interpretation: Normal sinus rhythm

27. Rate: 90
    Rhythm: Irregular
    P wave: Present and upright
    PRI: 0.16 seconds
    QRS: 0.04 seconds
    Interpretation: Sinus rhythm with PACs

28. Rate: 60
    Rhythm: Irregular
    P wave: Present and upright
    PRI: 0.16 seconds
    QRS: 0.04 seconds
    Interpretation: Sinus Rhythm with Sinus arrest

29. Rate: A
    Rhythm: A
    P wave: A
    PRI: A
    QRS: A
    Interpretation: Asystole

30. Rate: I
    Rhythm: I
    P wave: I
    PRI: I
    QRS: I
    Interpretation: Ventricular fibrillation (coarse)

31. Rate: 90
    Rhythm: Irregular (due to premature complexes)
    P wave: Present and upright for sinus beats
    PRI: 0.16 seconds
    QRS: 0.04 seconds
    Interpretation: Sinus rhythm with PACs (premature atrial complexes)

32. Rate: 120
Rhythm: Regular
P wave: Present; follow QRS complexes
PRI: I
QRS: 0.06 seconds
Interpretation: Junctional tachycardia

33. Rate: 70
Rhythm: Irregular
P wave: Present and upright (for sinus beats)
PRI: 0.12 seconds
QRS: 0.04 seconds
Interpretation: Sinus rhythm with unifocal PVCs

34. Rate: 70
Rhythm: Irregular
P wave: Present and upright (for sinus beats)
PRI: 0.16 seconds
QRS: 0.04 seconds (sinus beats)
Interpretation: Sinus rhythm with ventricular bigeminy

35. Rate: 80
Rhythm: Atrial—regular; ventricular—regular
P wave: Present and upright
PRI: Variable
QRS: 0.08 seconds
Interpretation: Third-degree (complete) heart block

36. Rate: I
Rhythm: Irregular
P wave: A
PRI: A
QRS: I
Interpretation: R on T phenomenon

37. Rate: 50
Rhythm: Essentially regular
P wave: Varying morphology
PRI: 0.16 seconds
QRS: 0.08 seconds
Interpretation: Wandering atrial pacemaker (WAP)

38. Rate: 130
Rhythm: Regular
P wave: Present and upright
PRI: 0.12 seconds
QRS: 0.04 seconds
Interpretation: Sinus tachycardia

39. Rate: A
Rhythm: A
P wave: A
PRI: A
QRS: A
Interpretation: Ventricular fibrillation (shock delivered—end of strip)

40. Rate: 90
Rhythm: Irregularly irregular
P wave: A
PRI: I
QRS: 0.04 seconds
Interpretation: Atrial fibrillation

41. Rate: 180
Rhythm: Regular
P wave: A
PRI: A
QRS: 0.16 seconds
Interpretation: Ventricular tachycardia

42. Rate: 60
Rhythm: Irregular (due to premature complexes)
P wave: Present and upright (for sinus beats)
PRI: 0.14 seconds
QRS: 0.04 seconds
Interpretation: Sinus rhythm with unifocal PVCs

43. Rate: 80
Rhythm: Irregular (due to premature complex)
P wave: A
PRI: A
QRS: 0.06 seconds
Interpretation: Atrial fibrillation with 1 PAC

44. Rate: A
Rhythm: I
P wave: A
PRI: A
QRS: A
Interpretation: Ventricular fibrillation

45. Rate: 100
Rhythm: Regular
P wave: Present and upright
PRI: 0.16 seconds
QRS: 0.08 seconds
Interpretation: Sinus tachycardia with ST segment elevation

46. Rate: 40
Rhythm: Regular
P wave: Present and upright
PRI: 0.16 seconds
QRS: 0.06 seconds
Interpretation: Sinus bradycardia

47. Rate: 120
Rhythm: Regular
P wave: Present and upright
PRI: 0.18 seconds
QRS: 0.04 seconds
Interpretation: Sinus tachycardia

48. Rate: 40
Rhythm: Irregular
P wave: Present and upright
PRI: Progressively prolonging
QRS: 0.04 seconds
Interpretation: Second-degree heart block, Mobitz type I, Wenckebach

49. Rate: Atrial—70; ventricular—40
Rhythm: Atrial—regular; ventricular—regular
P wave: Present and upright
PRI: Variable
QRS: 0.06 seconds
Interpretation: Third-degree (complete) heart block

50. Rate: 40
Rhythm: Regular
P wave: A
PRI: A
QRS: 0.06 seconds
Interpretation: Junctional escape rhythm

51. Rate: A
Rhythm: A
P wave: A
PRI: A
QRS: A
Interpretation: Asystole

52. Rate: 70
Rhythm: Regular
P wave: Present and upright
PRI: 0.16 seconds
QRS: 0.10 seconds
Interpretation: Normal sinus rhythm

53. Rate: 78
Rhythm: Regular
P wave: A
PRI: A
QRS: 0.08 seconds
Interpretation: Ventricular paced rhythm

54. Rate: 72
Rhythm: Regular
P wave: Inverted
PRI: 0.08 seconds
QRS: 0.04 seconds
Interpretation: Junctional rhythm

55. Rate: A
Rhythm: Irregular
P wave: A
PRI: A
QRS: A
Interpretation: Ventricular fibrillation

56. Rate: 80
     Rhythm: Regular
     P wave: Present and upright
     PRI: 0.16 seconds
     QRS: 0.08 seconds
     Interpretation: Normal sinus rhythm

57. Rate: 80
     Rhythm: Irregular
     P wave: Present and upright except with ectopic complexes
     PRI: 0.16 seconds
     QRS: 0.08 seconds
     Interpretation: Sinus rhythm with unifocal premature ventricular complexes

58. Rate: 70
     Rhythm: Irregular
     P wave: Present and upright except for ectopic beats
     PRI: 0.24 seconds
     QRS: 0.04 seconds
     Interpretation: First-degree heart block, ventricular bigeminy

59. Rate: 30
     Rhythm: Regular
     P wave: A
     PRI: A
     QRS: 0.10 seconds
     Interpretation: Idioventricular rhythm

60. Rate: I
     Rhythm: Irregular
     P wave: A
     PRI: A
     QRS: > 0.12 seconds
     Interpretation: Ventricular tachycardia with short run of V fib

61. Rate: 10
     Rhythm: Irregular
     P wave: A
     PRI: A
     QRS: 0.04 seconds
     Interpretation: Sinus arrest (5.6 seconds)

62. Rate: I
     Rhythm: Irregular
     P wave: A
     PRI: A
     QRS: 0.04 seconds (sinus complexes), then 0.12 seconds in ectopic complexes
     Interpretation: Frequent PVCs with run of V tach; atrial fibrillation

63. Rate: 80 (atrial)
     Rhythm: Regular
     P wave: Present and upright
     PRI: I
     QRS: A
     Interpretation: Ventricular standstill

64. Rate: Atrial—100; Ventricular—40
    Rhythm: Regular
    P wave: Present and upright
    PRI: Variable
    QRS: 0.10 seconds
    Interpretation: Third-degree heart block

65. Rate: 70
    Rhythm: Regular
    P wave: A
    PRI: A
    QRS: 0.04 seconds
    Interpretation: Atrial paced rhythm

66. Rate: 80
    Rhythm: Irregular
    P wave: Present and upright
    PRI: 0.16 seconds
    QRS: 0.04 seconds
    Interpretation: Sinus rhythm with multifocal PVCs

67. Rate: 110
    Rhythm: Irregular
    P wave: A
    PRI: A
    QRS: 0.04 seconds
    Interpretation: Atrial fibrillation

68. Rate: 80
    Rhythm: Irregular
    P wave: Present and upright
    PRI: 0.16 seconds
    QRS: 0.04 seconds
    Interpretation: Normal sinus rhythm with a run of VT

69. Rate: 70
    Rhythm: Regularly irregular
    P wave: Present and upright in normal complexes except ectopic beats
    PRI: 0.16 seconds
    QRS: 0.04 seconds
    Interpretation: NSR with ventricular bigeminy

70. Rate: 100
    Rhythm: Regularly irregular
    P wave: Present and upright in normal complexes except ectopic beats
    PRI: 0.16 seconds
    QRS: 0.04 seconds
    Interpretation: NSR with ventricular trigeminy

71. Rate: 190
    Rhythm: Regular
    P wave: None
    PRI: None
    QRS: 0.20 seconds
    Interpretation: Ventricular tachycardia

72. Rate: Atrial—110; ventricular—30
　　 Rhythm: Regular
　　 P wave: Present and Upright
　　 PRI: 0.14 seconds
　　 QRS: 0.04 seconds
　　 Interpretation: Mobitz Type II, second-degree heart block

73. Rate: 80
　　 Rhythm: Regular
　　 P wave: Flutter waves
　　 PRI: I
　　 QRS: 0.04 seconds
　　 Interpretation: Atrial flutter—4:1 ratio

74. Rate: 80
　　 Rhythm: Regular
　　 P wave: Present and upright
　　 PRI: 0.16 seconds
　　 QRS: 0.08 seconds
　　 Interpretation: Normal sinus rhythm (ST elevation)

75. Rate: 130
　　 Rhythm: Irregularly irregular
　　 P wave: I
　　 PRI: I
　　 QRS: 0.08 seconds
　　 Interpretation: Atrial fibrillation

76. Rate: 120
　　 Rhythm: Regular
　　 P wave: Present and upright
　　 PRI: 0.16 seconds
　　 QRS: 0.04 seconds
　　 Interpretation: Sinus tachycardia

77. Rate: 40
　　 Rhythm: Regular
　　 P wave: Inverted
　　 PRI: 0.08 seconds
　　 QRS: 0.04 seconds
　　 Interpretation: Junctional escape rhythm

78. Rate: 70
　　 Rhythm: Irregular
　　 P wave: Present and upright
　　 PRI: 0.20 seconds
　　 QRS: 0.06 seconds
　　 Interpretation: Sinus rhythm with PAC

79. Rate: 90
　　 Rhythm: Regular
　　 P wave: Present and upright
　　 PRI: 0.24 seconds
　　 QRS: 0.08 seconds
　　 Interpretation: First-degree block

80. Rate: I
      Rhythm: Irregular
      P wave: A
      PRI: A
      QRS: I
      Interpretation: Ventricular fibrillation

81. Rate: 60
      Rhythm: Irregular
      P wave: Present and upright
      PRI: Progressively prolonging
      QRS: 0.04 seconds
      Interpretation: Second-degree block Type I, Wenckebach

82. Rate: 80
      Rhythm: Irregular
      P wave: Present and upright with normal complexes
      PRI: 0.16 seconds
      QRS: 0.04 seconds
      Interpretation: NSR with multifocal PVCs

83. Rate: 70
      Rhythm: Regular
      P wave: Present and upright
      PRI: 0.16 seconds
      QRS: 0.04 seconds
      Interpretation: Second-degree heart block Mobitz Type II (2:1 ratio)

84. Rate: 90
      Rhythm: Irregular
      P wave: Present and upright in normal complexes
      PRI: 0.12 seconds
      QRS: 0.08 seconds
      Interpretation: NSR into a ventricular bigeminy

85. Rate: 20
      Rhythm: Regular
      P wave: I
      PRI: I
      QRS: 0.16 seconds
      Interpretation: Idioventricular Rhythm

86. Rate: 100
      Rhythm: Regular
      P wave: Present and upright
      PRI: 0.16 seconds
      QRS: 0.04 seconds
      Interpretation: Normal sinus rhythm with ST elevation

87. Rate: 170
      Rhythm: Irregular
      P wave: Present and upright
      PRI: 0.20 seconds
      QRS: 0.04 seconds
      Interpretation: Sinus tachycardia (post shock with initial ventricular ectopic beats)

88. Rate: 70
Rhythm: Irregular
P wave: A
PRI: A
QRS: 0.10 (paced complexes)
Interpretation: Paced rhythm with two failure to capture beats

89. Rate: 40
Rhythm: Regular
P wave: Present and upright
PRI: 0.12 seconds
QRS: 0.04 seconds
Interpretation: Sinus bradycardia

90. Rate: 100
Rhythm: Irregular
P wave: Present and upright
PRI: 0.12 seconds
QRS: 0.04 seconds
Interpretation: Sinus rhythm with multifocal PVCs

91. Rate: 100
Rhythm: Irregular
P wave: Present and upright
PRI: 0.20 seconds
QRS: 0.04 seconds
Interpretation: Sinus rhythm with unifocal PVCs

92. Rate: 160
Rhythm: Regular
P wave: A
PRI: A
QRS: 0.26 seconds
Interpretation: Ventricular tachycardia

93. Rate: 100
Rhythm: Irregular
P wave: Present and upright
PRI: 0.12 seconds
QRS 0.04 seconds
Interpretation: Sinus rhythm with ventricular bigeminy

94. Rate: 60
Rhythm: Irregular
P wave: Present and upright
PRI: 0.16 seconds
QRS: 0.04 seconds
Interpretation: Sinus rhythm with a PAC

95. Rate: 180
Rhythm: Regular
P wave: Present and upright
PRI: 0.12 seconds
QRS: 0.04 seconds
Interpretation: Sinus tachycardia

96. Rate: 80
      Rhythm: Irregular
      P wave: Present and upright
      PRI: 0.20 seconds
      QRS: 0.04 seconds
      Interpretation: Sinus dysrhythmia with frequent unifocal PVCs

97. Rate: 80
      Rhythm: Regular
      P wave: Present and upright
      PRI: 0.14 seconds
      QRS: 0.04 seconds
      Interpretation: Normal sinus rhythm

98. Rate: 60
      Rhythm: Regular
      P wave: A
      PRI: A
      QRS: 0.04 seconds
      Interpretation: Junctional escape rhythm

99. Rate: 100
      Rhythm: Regular
      P wave: Present and upright
      PRI: 0.12 seconds
      QRS: 0.04 seconds
      Interpretation: Normal sinus rhythm

100. Rate: 150
      Rhythm: Regular
      P wave: Present and upright
      PRI: 0.14 seconds
      QRS: I (due to ST elevation)
      Interpretation: Sinus tachycardia with ST elevation

Glossary

A

absolute refractory period stage of cell activity in which the cardiac cell cannot spontaneously depolarize

accelerated idioventricular rhythm (AIVR) occurs when the rate of the ectopic pacemaker in an idioventricular rhythm exceeds 40 BPM

accelerated junctional rhythm increased automaticity in the AV junction, causing the junction to discharge impulses at a rate faster than its intrinsic rate

accessory pathway irregular muscle connection between the atria and ventricles that bypasses the AV node

acetylcholine the chemical neurotransmitter for the parasympathetic nervous system

acute myocardial infarction (heart attack) resulting from a prolonged lack of blood flow to a portion of the myocardial tissue and results in a lack of oxygen

afterload the resistance against which the heart must pump

agonal when the rate of an IVR rhythm falls below 20 BPM, the rhythm may be called agonal

angina pectoris pain that results from a reduction in blood supply to myocardial tissue

anion an ion with a negative charge

aortic valve the semilunar valve located between the left ventricle and the trunk of the aorta

arteries thick-walled and muscular blood vessels that function under high pressure to convey blood from the heart out to the rest of the body

artifact EKG waveforms from sources outside the heart

artificial pacemaker a device that substitutes for the normal pacemaker cells of the heart's electrical conduction system

atherosclerosis narrowed coronary arterial walls, secondary to fatty deposits

atrial dysrhythmias the group of dysrhythmias produced when the SA node fails to generate an impulse and the atrial tissues or areas in the internodal pathways initiate an impulse

atrial fibrillation when multiple disorganized ectopic atrial foci generate electrical activity at a very rapid rate (atrial rate varies from 350–750 BPM)

atrial flutter when a single irritable site in the atria initiates many electrical impulses at a rapid rate, characterized by the presence of regular atrial activity with a picket-fence or sawtooth pattern

atrial kick the final phase of diastole, atrial contraction forces remaining blood into the ventricles; provides 15 to 30 percent of ventricular filling

atrioventricular (AV) node located on the floor of the right atrium near the opening of the coronary sinus and just above the tricuspid valve; at the level of the AV node, the electrical activity is delayed approximately 0.05 seconds

atrium upper chamber of the heart

automaticity the ability of cardiac pacemaker cells to generate their own electrical impulses spontaneously without external (or nervous) stimulation

autonomic nervous system (ANS) regulates functions of the body that are involuntary, or not under conscious control

AV junction the region where the AV node joins the bundle of His

B

Bachmann's bundle a subdivision of the anterior internodal tract, conducts electrical activity from the SA node to the left atrium

baseline the straight line seen on an EKG strip; it represents the beginning and end point of all waves

Beck's triad muffled heart sounds, JVD, and narrowing pulse pressure

bipolar leads have one positive electrode and one negative electrode

bradycardia heart rate of less than 60 BPM

bundle branches two main branches, the right bundle branch and the left bundle branch, conduct electrical activity from the bundle of His down to the Purkinje network

bundle of His the conduction pathway that leads out of the AV node and is also traditionally referred to as the *common bundle*

C

capillaries tiny blood vessels that allow for the exchange of oxygen, nutrients, and waste products between the blood and body tissues; "connectors" between arteries and veins

capture noted by the presence of a spike and wide QRS complexes, the presence of an adequate carotid pulse and blood pressure, and an increased level of consciousness

cardiac cycle the actual time sequence between ventricular contraction and ventricular relaxation

cardiac output the amount of blood pumped by the left ventricle in 1 min

cardiac tamponade an excess accumulation of fluid in the pericardial sac

cardiogenic shock when left ventricular function is so severely compromised that the heart can no longer meet the metabolic requirements of the body

cardioversion refers to the process of the passage of an electric current through the heart during a specific part of the cardiac cycle for the purpose of terminating certain kinds of dysrhythmias

cation an ion with a positive charge

chest pain is the most common presenting symptom of cardiac disease, as well as the most common complaint by patients

chordae tendineae fine chords of dense connective tissue that attach to papillary muscles in the wall of the ventricles

circulation movement through a course (the body) which leads back to the initial point (the heart)

compensatory pause a pause that occurs after an ectopic beat in which the SA node is unaffected and the cadence of the heart is uninterrupted

conductivity the ability of cardiac cells to receive an electrical stimulus and then transmit it to other cardiac cells

congestive heart failure (CHF) when the heart's stroke volume becomes severely diminished and causes an overload of fluid in systemic tissues

contractility (also referred to as rhythmicity) is the ability of cardiac cells to shorten and cause cardiac muscle contraction in response to an electrical stimulus

coronary arteries two main arteries that arise from the trunk of the aorta and function to carry oxygenated blood throughout the myocardium

coronary circulation is the process by which oxygenated blood is distributed throughout the heart muscle

coronary sinus (also referred to as the Great Cardiac Vein) a short trunk that serves to receive deoxygenated blood from the veins of the myocardium

coronary sulcus the atrioventricular groove that surrounds the outside of the heart and divides the atria from the ventricles

D

defibrillation the process of passing an electrical current through a fibrillating heart to depolarize the cells and allow them to repolarize uniformly, thus restoring an organized/normal rhythm after the onset of fibrillation

demand, or synchronous, pacemaker generates electrical impulses when the patient's heart rate falls below a predetermined rate

diaphoresis profuse sweating

diastole is synonymous with ventricular relaxation

dyspnea labored breathing

dysrhythmias abnormal heart rhythms

E

EKG waveforms a wave or waveform recorded on an EKG strip refers to movement away from the baseline or isoelectric line and is represented as a positive deflection (above the isoelectric line) or as a negative deflection (below the isoelectric line)

electrocardiogram graphic representation of the electrical activity of the heart

electrocardiograph machine used to record the electrocardiogram

electrode an adhesive pad that contains conductive gel and is designed to be attached to the patient's skin

electrolyte a substance or compound whose molecules dissociate into charged components, or ions, when placed in water, producing positively and negatively charged ions

endocardium the innermost layer of the heart; composed of thin connective tissue

epicardium the smooth outer surface of the heart

excitability the ability of cardiac cells to respond to an electrical stimulus, a characteristic shared by all cardiac cells

F

first-degree heart block the most usual form of block, resulting from excessive conduction delay in the AV node

fixed-rate, or asynchronous, pacemaker programmed to deliver electrical impulses at a constant selected rate

G

generator controls the rate and strength of each electrical impulse

H

heart blocks electrical conduction system disorders

heart failure the inability of the myocardium to meet the cardiac output demands of the body

heart rate the number of contractions, or beats, per minute of the heart

heart rhythm the sequential beating of the heart as a result of the generation of electrical impulses

hemodynamically stable refers to a patient who presents with a normal blood pressure (normotensive), absence of chest pain, and no notable change in mental status

hemodynamically unstable refers to a patient who presents with hypotension (low blood pressure), chest pain, shortness of breath, and changes in mental status

hypovolemia decreased blood volume

hypoxia low oxygen level

I

idioventricular rhythms (IVRs) (also called ventricular escape rhythms) result when the discharge rate of higher pacemakers become less than that of the ventricles or when impulses from higher pacemakers fail to reach the ventricles

inferior vena cava collects blood from the rest of the body

internodal tracts distribute the electrical impulse throughout the atria and transmit the impulse from the SA node to the AV node

interpolated beat occurs when a PVC falls between two sinus beats without interfering with the rhythm

J

J point the point where the QRS complex meets the ST segment

junctional escape rhythm when the SA node fails to generate an impulse or if the rate of impulse generation falls below that of the AV node, then the AV node will assume the role of the pacemaker; the resulting rhythm is called a junctional escape rhythm

junctional rhythms rhythms that are initiated in the area of the AV junction

junctional tachycardia rhythm a rhythm arising from the AV junctional tissue at a rate of 100 to 180 BPM

junctional tachycardia when the junctional firing rate exceeds 100 BPM

L

lead a pair of electrodes such as chest Lead I, II, MCL

lead wires relay the electrical impulse from the generator to the myocardium

leads electrodes connected to the monitor or EKG machine by wires

left ventricular failure when a patient's left ventricle ceases to function in an adequate capacity as to sustain sufficient systemic cardiac output

M

mediastinum the central section of the thorax (chest cavity)

mitral (or bicuspid) valve similar in structure to the tricuspid valve but has only two cusps and is located between the left atrium and the left ventricle

morphology shape of the PVC

multifocal PVCs with different shapes that originate from different sites within the ventricles

multifocal atrial tachycardia (MAT) the rhythm created when the rate of the wandering atrial pacemaker rhythm reaches 100 BPM or greater

myocardial ischemia decreased supply of oxygenated blood to the heart

myocardial working cells responsible for generating the physical contraction of the heart muscle

myocardium the thick middle layer of the heart composed primarily of cardiac muscle cells and responsible for the heart's ability to contract

N

neuropathy inability to perceive pain due to diseases of the nerves

nitroglycerin causes dilation of the blood vessels that consequently reduces the workload of the heart

noncompensatory pause the pause that occurs after an ectopic beat, when the SA node is depolarized

nonsustained rhythm a run of VT that lasts for less than 30 seconds

norepinephrine the chemical neurotransmitter for the sympathetic nervous system

normal sinus rhythm the rhythm that occurs when the SA node has generated an impulse that followed the normal pathway of the electrical conduction system and led to atrial and ventricular depolarization

O

oxygen the most important drug that any patient with chest pain can receive

P

P wave represents depolarization of the left and right atria

pacemaker spike the EKG wave produced by an artificial pacemaker

palpitations a sensation that the heart is skipping beats and/or beating rapidly

parasympathetic nervous system regulates the calmer (rest and digest) functions

paroxysmal refers to a sudden onset or cessation or both

paroxysmal junctional tachycardia (PJT) rhythm a junctional tachycardia rhythm that is observed to begin or end abruptly

paroxysmal rhythm a rhythm observed to start or end abruptly

pericarditis an inflammation of the serous pericardium

pericardium closed, two-layered sac that surrounds the heart; "potential space" between the visceral and parietal layers of the pericardium holds a small amount of pericardial fluid (approximately 10–20 cc)

peripheral vascular resistance (PVR) the amount of opposition to blood flow offered by the arterioles

permanent pacemakers implanted inside the patient's upper left chest (most commonly) and are left in place

PR interval measures the time intervals from the onset of atrial contraction to the onset of ventricular contraction

preload the pressure in the ventricles at the end of diastole

premature atrial contraction (PAC) a single, electrical impulse that originates outside the SA node in the atria

premature junctional contractions (PJCs) initiate from a single site in the AV junction and arise earlier than the next anticipated complex of the underlying rhythm

premature ventricular complex a single, ectopic (out-of-place) complex that occurs earlier than the next expected complex and arises from an irritable site in the ventricles

Prinzmetal's angina or **vasospastic angina** form of angina that can occur when the coronary arteries experience spasms and constrict

pulmonary circulation when blood leaves the heart through the right ventricle and travels into the pulmonary artery to the lungs and back through the pulmonary veins to the left atrium

pulmonary edema backup of blood in the pulmonary system that causes plasma to mix with and displace alveolar air

pulmonic valve the semilunar valve located between the right ventricle and the pulmonary artery

pulseless electrical activity (PEA) the absence of a palpable pulse and myocardial muscle activity with the presence of organized electrical activity (excluding VT or VF) on the cardiac monitor

pulsus paradoxus evidenced by a systolic blood pressure that drops more than 10–15 mmHg during inspiration

Purkinje's network a network of fibers that carries electrical impulses directly to ventricular muscle cells

Q

QRS complex consists of the Q, R, and S waves and represents the conduction of the electrical impulse from the bundle of His throughout the ventricular muscle, or ventricular depolarization; represents the depolarization (or contraction) of the ventricles

R

rapid ventricular response a ventricular rate of 100 to 150 BPM

reentry the reactivation of myocardial tissue for a second or subsequent time by the same electrical impulse

relative refractory period the period when repolarization is almost complete, and the cardiac cell can be stimulated to contract prematurely if the stimulus is much stronger than normal

retrograde contrary (or opposite of) to the normal expected path of movement

rhythm strip or EKG strip the printed record of the electrical activity of the heart

right heart failure when the right ventricle ceases to function properly, causing an increase in pressure within the right atrium, thus forcing the blood backward into the systemic venous system

S

SA node commonly referred to as the primary pacemaker of the heart because it normally depolarizes more rapidly than any other part of the conduction system

salvos another name given to a run or grouping of three or more PVCs in a row

second-degree AV block, Mobitz type I, or Wenckenbach the progressive prolongation of the electrical impulse delay at the AV node, which produces an increase in the length of the PR interval

second-degree AV block, or Mobitz type II a more serious dysrhythmia that occurs when there is an intermittent interruption in the electrical conduction system near or below the AV junction

semilunar valves serve to prevent the backflow of blood into the ventricles and each valve contains three semilunar (or moon-shaped) cusps

sensing is simply the capability of a pacemaker to recognize inherent electrical conduction system activity

sinus arrest rhythm when the sinus node fails to discharge, the absence of a PQRST interval is noted on the rhythm strip

sinus bradycardia in this rhythm, the SA node discharges impulses at a rate of less than 60 BPM

sinus dysrhythmia an irregular rhythm produced when the P-to-P intervals and the R-to-R intervals change with respirations

sinus tachycardia a variant of normal sinus rhythm; the rate is generally considered to be 100 to 160 BPM

site of origin rhythms are classified according to the heart structure or structures in which they begin

slow ventricular response a ventricular rate of less than 60 BPM

specialized group responsible for controlling the rate and rhythm of the heart by coordinating regular depolarization and are found in the electrical conduction system of the heart

ST segment begins with the end of the QRS complex and ends with the onset of the T wave

stable, or predictable angina a particular activity may elicit chest pain

Starling's Law of the heart more the myocardial fibers are stretched, up to a certain point, the more forceful the subsequent contraction will be

stroke volume the volume of blood pumped out of one ventricle of the heart in a single beat or contraction

superior vena cava drains blood from the head and neck

supraventricular above the ventricles

supraventricular tachycardia (SVT) a general term that encompasses all fast (tachy-) dysrhythmias in which the heart rate is greater than 100 BPM

sustained rhythm a rhythm that lasts for more than 30 seconds

sympathetic nervous system responsible for preparation of the body for physical activity (fight or flight)

systemic circulation the circulation of blood as it leaves the left ventricle and travels through the arteries, capillaries, and veins of the entire body system and back to the primary receptacle of the heart (the right atrium)

systole, or ventricular systole is consistent with the simultaneous contraction of the ventricles

T

T wave produced by ventricular repolarization or relaxation; represents ventricular repolarization and follows the ST segment

tachycardia heart rate greater than 100 BPM

temporary pacemakers used to sustain a patient's heart rate in emergent situations

third-degree AV block (complete) the most serious type of heart block; the atria and ventricles are completely blocked or separated from each other electrically at or below the AV node; ventricular rate will most commonly be between 20 and 40 BPM

threshold refers to the point at which a stimulus will produce a cell response

thrombus formation the most common cause of myocardial infarction; results in blockage of the coronary artery

tissue perfusion refers to gas exchange within the alveolar capillary membranes in the lungs

torsades de pointes similar to ventricular tachycardia; morphology of QRS complexes show variations in width and shape; life-threatening dysrhythmia

transcutaneous pacing (TCP) commonly called external cardiac pacing, consists of two large electrode pads, which are most commonly placed in an anterior-posterior position on the patient's chest to conduct electrical impulses through the skin to the heart

transvenous pacing (through a vein) a lead wire is inserted through the skin and threaded into a large vein leading into the right side of the heart and controlled by an external power source

tricuspid valve named for its three cusps; located between the right atrium and the right ventricle

U

unifocal PVCs that are alike in appearance

unstable angina pain not elicited by activity that most commonly occurs while the patient is at rest; also referred to as "preinfarctional" angina

V

vagal maneuvers methods utilized to stimulate baroreceptors (located in the internal carotid and aortic arch); when these receptors are stimulated, the vagus nerves release acetylcholine, resulting in a slowing of the heart rate

veins blood vessels that carry blood back to the heart, operate under low pressure, and are relatively thin walled

ventricle lower chamber of the heart

ventricular asystole the absence of all ventricular activity; also called cardiac standstill or asystole; the absence of all cardiac electrical activity

ventricular fibrillation (VF, V fib) is a fatal dysrhythmia that occurs as a result of multiple weak ectopic foci in the ventricles; there is no coordinated atrial or ventricular contraction and no palpable pulse

ventricular tachycardia (VT, V tach) rhythm in which three or more PVCs arise in sequence at a rate of greater than 100 BPM; commonly overrides the normal pacemaker of the heart

W

wandering atrial pacemaker (WAP) rhythms occur when pacemaker sites wander, or travel, from the SA node to other pacemaker sites in the atria, the internodal pathways, or the AV node

Wolff-Parkinson-White (WPW) syndrome preexcitation syndrome and atrioventricular conduction disorder characterized by two AV conduction pathways and is often identified by a characteristic delta wave seen on an electrocardiogram at the beginning of the QRS complex

Index

W